ABDURAHMAN SHERALIYEV

Response of embryonic, maternal liver mitochondrial membranes

ABDURAHMAN SHERALIYEV

Response of embryonic, maternal liver mitochondrial membranes

and placenta on the effects of butifos

ScienciaScripts

Imprint

Cover image: www.ingimage.com

This book is a translation from the original published under ISBN 978-620-7-45510-2.

Publisher:
Sciencia Scripts
is a trademark of
Dodo Books Indian Ocean Ltd. and OmniScriptum S.R.L publishing group

120 High Road, East Finchley, London, N2 9ED, United Kingdom
Str. Armeneasca 28/1, office 1, Chisinau MD-2012, Republic of Moldova, Europe
Printed at: see last page
ISBN: 978-620-7-78989-4

Contents

INTRODUCTION

Increasing crop yields is one of the most important ways of solving the food programme of our independent country. The large-scale use of pesticides of various spectrums of action plays a major role in this endeavour. Decisions by the Government and the Head of State provide for a further increase in the production of mineral fertilisers, chemical means of controlling weeds, pests and pathogens of agricultural plants. In particular, organophosphorus compounds are increasingly being used in many areas of human activity. They are used on a large scale in agriculture as pesticides, as well as in various technological processes in industry.

Such diverse practical use of organophosphorus compounds in the national economy, while maintaining the trend of further growth of their production and use, the presence of residual quantities of applied pesticides in agricultural products, as well as the specificity of the methods of treatment of agricultural objects with them dictate the need for a thorough study of the effect of organophosphorus compounds on biochemical and physiological processes occurring in the organism of animals and humans.

The approach to studying the mechanism of pesticide action on warm-blooded organisms is diverse and complex. In particular, the effect of pesticides on intrauterine development, as well as identification of their teratogenic and embryotropic properties, attracts wide attention. The action of teratogens can be manifested at different levels of organisation of a living organism, in changes in various aspects of metabolism in the cell (Barilyak, Kalinovskaya, 1977,1979; Dyban, 1965; Wilson, 1973).However, the significance of these metabolic disturbances of the intrauterine foetus in the occurrence of various anatomical and functional anomalies has not been fully deciphered. The action of some teratogenic substances has been studied mainly at the organ and tissue level, and their effects at the level of cell membranes during embryogenesis are much less well studied.

Meanwhile, studies conducted at the cellular and subcellular levels make it possible to characterise the effect of a particular pesticide on a specific process localised in certain structures, which is particularly important for elucidating the primary stages of interaction between a foreign substance and cell components.

In biochemical analysis of the toxic effect of pesticides, a special place is occupied by their influence on structural and functional properties of subcellular formations and, first of all, on mitochondrial membranes. According to a number of authors (Rotenberg, 1980; Abo-Khatwa, Holiingworth, 1974), based on analyses of the effects of many dozens of pesticides, mitochondria are the most probable targets of their action.

The main functions of mitochondria are related to the ATP-synthetase complex and redox enzymes located on the inner mitochondrial membrane. Mitochondria play a predominant role in the energy metabolism of animal tissue cells at all stages of ontogenesis, including intrauterine development. The morphology of mitochondria during embryonic development has been studied in detail, but data on the activity of mitochondrial enzymes during organ growth and differentiation are contradictory (Sentyurova, 1975; Greenfeld, Boell, 1968; Makler, 1971).

It has been shown that the effect of pesticides on the embryo depends on the dose, duration of drug administration, and gestational age. However, such important issues as the functioning of membrane-bound enzymes of mitochondria of differentiating tissues under the action of pesticides are also insufficiently studied. In connection with the above, it was of undoubted interest to find out the state of oxidative phosphorylation, activity of some polyenzyme systems, phospholipid composition and some other properties of mitochondrial membranes of liver mitochondria of embryos, maternal organism and placenta under the action of pesticides.

Within this goal, the following tasks were to be accomplished:

1) to study the effect of butifos, a defoliant widely used in cotton growing, one of the representatives of organophosphorus pesticides, on respiration and oxidative phosphorylation of mitochondria in the liver of embryos, maternal organism and placenta;

2) to investigate the effect of butifos on the activity of NAD.H-oxidase, succinatoxidase and cytochrome c-oxidase of liver mitochondria of embryos, maternal organism and placenta;

3) to investigate the effect of butifos on the phospholipid and protein composition of mitochondrial membranes of liver mitochondria of embryos, maternal organism and placenta.

In connection with the solution of these problems, we have established:

administration of butifos to pregnant rabbits on the 23rd day of pregnancy slightly increases the efficiency of the energy conversion system in the liver mitochondria of pregnant rabbits, but on the 30th day of pregnancy the effect of butifos is characterised by a decrease in the value of parameters characterising the oxidative phosphorylation of maternal liver mitochondria;

mitochondria isolated from the placenta of experimental groups of animals are characterised by an increased rate of electron transfer along the respiratory chain. The respiration of mitochondria in metabolic states V4* and V4 is especially markedly increased, which leads to a decrease in the value of respiratory control. However, mitochondria isolated from the placenta on the 30th day of pregnancy, under the influence of butifos have a reduced rate of succinate oxidation, especially in the V4 state. As a result of butifos administration in embryo liver mitochondria on the 23rd day of development, there is an increase in the rate of electron transport along the respiratory chain and an improvement in drug conjugation, and on the 30th day - a decrease in the parameters of oxidative phosphorylation;

the activity of polyenzyme systems of the respiratory chain mitochondria of embryo liver increases under the influence of butifos, while that of maternal liver mitochondria and placenta decreases;

at a single injection of butifos in mitochondria of liver of embryos and maternal organism there is an increase in the content of phosphatidylethanolamine, phosphatidylcholine, phosphatidylserine, phosphatidic acid and a decrease in cardiolipin, sphingomyelin, lysophos-fatidylcholine, lysophosphatidylethanolamine and lysocardiolipin. At the same time in placenta mitochondria the content of phosphatidylethanolamine, phosphatidylserine, phosphatidylcholine and phosphatidic acid decreases, at the same time the concentration of cardiolipin, phosphatidylinositol, sphingomyelin and lysophosphatidylethanolamine increases.

Chapter I

LITERATURE REVIEW

I.I. Structure and functions of mitochondria in embryonic development.

1.1.1 Mitochondrial membrane structure and respiratory chain composition.

Mitochondria consist of outer and inner membranes, their shape and size are tissue-specific and change during development (Bovyagin, 1974; Green and Fleischer, 1964; Green and Goldberger, 1968; Le- ninger, 1966, 1974; Sjoatrand, 1978).

Thanks to different methodological approaches in electron microscopy, the ultrastructural organisation of mitochondrial membranes has been studied. In the central region of mitochondrial membranes there is a continuous bilipid layer, in the hydrophobic region of which hydrophobic peptide regions of enzymes and glycoproteins are immersed from the matrix and intermembrane space (Borovyagin, 1974).

Sjostrand (1978) developed original methods of preparation of preparations for electron microscopic analysis and proposed a scheme of biomembrane structure. The fundamental differences in the ultrastructural organisation of mitochondrial outer and inner membranes were revealed.

The 150 A thick mitochondrial inner membrane consists of a three-dimensional protein-lipid structure, with the lipid layer accounting for 1/3 of its thickness.

The outer and inner membranes of mitochondria differ considerably in chemical composition, structural, morphological and functional properties (Archakov, 1971; Parsons, 1967; Smolyetal., 1970; Eraster, Kuylenstiema, 1970; Lee, 1971).

The inner membrane of mitochondria belongs to the number of "conjugating biomembranes", i.e. it has a well-defined function. It contains the enzymes of the respiratory chain and phosphorylation (Lehninger, 1966; O'Brien, Matlid, 1973). In the laboratory of Schnaitman (Schnaitmanetai., 1968) and other researchers (Poglazov, 1973; (Scholte, 1973; Maisterrenaetal., 1974), reliable results have been obtained from which it follows that monoamine oxidase,NAD.H-cytochrome-s-reductase (rotenone-insensitive), NAD.H-oxidase, kynurenine hydroxylase.

All proteins of the outer membrane and mitochondrial matrix, as well as most of the proteins of the inner mitochondrial membrane, are synthesised outside mitochondria. The polypeptide chains synthesised in mitochondria are relatively hydrophobic and firmly bound to the membrane (Birchmeier, 1977; Felter, stani, 1978). Such a protein has been isolated in lipid-free form and labelled as a structural protein (Kadenbach, 1967).

The mitochondrial membrane system is not only the structural basis of mitochondria, but also contains highly organised enzymatic ensembles that integrate numerous processes of cellular metabolism (Lehninger, 1966; Skulachev, 1969).

The main function of the mitochondrial respiratory chain is the oxidation of NAD.H and succinate by a system of electron-transferring molecules. The substrates enter the Krebs cycle and give hydrogen atoms to nico-tinamidadenine dinucleotide molecules or flavoprotein in the case of succinate (Fig. I). The reduced NAD-H is oxidised by the mitochondrial respiratory chain in several steps (the first is between NADH dehydrogenase and Q_{10} , the second is between cytochromes *y* and c, and the third is between cytochrome c and oxygen), which is accompanied by accumulation of oxidation energy and ATP synthesis (Lehninger, 1966,1974; Skulachev, 1969; Green and Goldberger, 1968; Racker, 1979).

NAD.N.
Suk cynate

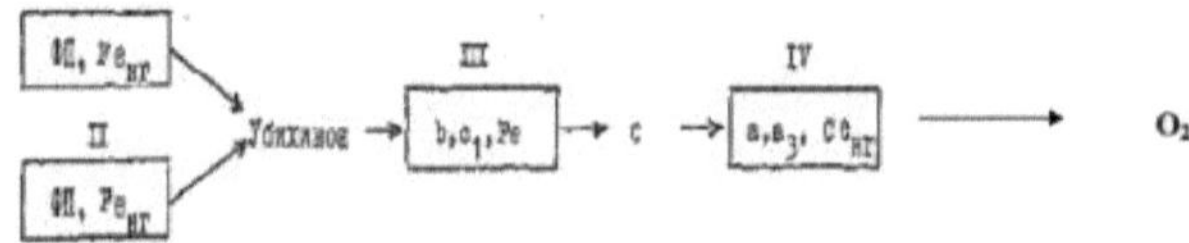

Fig.1. according to V.P. Skulachev (1969)

In fact, ATP formation is inseparably coupled with the oxidation process, so on firmly coupled preparations of mitochondria in the absence of ADP and $F_{н}$ respiration practically ceases. For each molecule of NAD.H that is oxidised by molecular oxygen, 3 molecules of ATP are formed; the P/0 (or ADP/0) coefficient for this process, reflecting its efficiency, is 3, and for succinate oxidation it is 2.

From a functional point of view, the following segments of the mitochondrial respiratory chain can be distinguished (Fig. I).

1. Oxidation of NAD.H and reduction of coenzyme Q.

The polyenzyme system that catalyses the catalytic acceleration of this process is called complex I. This complex with high activity was first obtained by Hatefietai in 1962. Subsequently, this complex was separated into flavoprotein and non-heme iron protein (Hatefietai.,1962). Purified NAD.H-dehydrogenase does not contain flavin. It is a component of NADH oxidase of the respiratory chain (Dancey and Shapiro, 1976). The reaction catalysed by isolated NAD.H-dehydrogenase is insensitive to rotenone, in contrast to intact mitochondria or submitochondrial particles, and its activation depends on the pH of the medium (Agureev et al., 1981).

2. Oxidation of succinate and reduction of coenzyme Q.

The succinatoxidase system occupies a special position among the energy-converting systems in the cell (Kondrashova, 1971; Vinogradov, 1982). The initial link of this system is the reaction of oxidation of succinic acid to fumaric acid, which is catalysed by succinate dehydrogenase. The activity of this enzyme can be altered by succinate, fumarate and phosphate. Succinate dehydrogenase is firmly associated with the inner mitochondrial membrane of animal cell mitochondria (Lehninger, 1974) and is thought to be located on the inner surface of the inner mitochondrial membrane (Ackreiietal.,1978).

3. Oxidation of reduced coenzyme by cytochrome c.

Complex Sh was isolated by Hatefietal., (1962). This is the most studied complex of the respiratory chain (Gavrikova et al., 1977; Weiss, Juchs, 1978). Its main components are cytochrome b cytochrome C'|I A non-heme iron protein. When studying cytochrome b,c1 cytochrome complex and its subunits, it was found that cytochrome c1 is the direct functional and structural partner of cytochrome b of mitochondrial cytochrome reductase.

Complex Sh contains an oxidation factor required for the reduction of cytochrome c by cytochrome b (Hishibayashietal., 1972). This factor is a labile protein giving an EPR signal of g= 1.90. Erecinckaetal., (1976) isolated and purified a cytochrome c1 complex which appears to contain equimolar amounts of cytochrome c1,b_{565} ,b_{562} iron and protein. Cytochrome ^^ is thought to be localised on the outer side of the membrane and cytochrome b_{562} on the inner side.

4. Oxidation of reduced cytochrome c with oxygen.

Cytochrome c-oxidase (complex 1U) is a subunit protein. It is assumed that a polypeptide with a molecular weight of 9500 is the precursor of the cytochrome c-oxidase subunit (Koioravetal., 1981).Complex 1U contains two spectrally distinct cytochromes, a and a_3 .Complex 1U is the end site of the respiratory chain and carries out electron transfer from the reduced cytochrome c. The catalytic function of cytochrome c is to transfer electron from cytochrome b and c1 complex to cytochrome c oxidase. Cytochrome oxidase subunits interact with phospholipids
mitochondrial membranes (Bissonetal, 1979). Cytochrome oxidase consists of2 groups of subunits (Sebaldetal., 1973; Poyton, Schatz, 1975; Hundt, Kadenback, 1977). The first of them is represented by less hydrophobic polypeptides, which are synthesised by the nuclear-cytoplasmic system and provide the catalytic function of the enzyme proper. The second group of polypeptides is characterised by increased hydrophobicity and is synthesised in mitochondria. A complete reconstruction of cytochrome oxidase (it consists of 8 protein subunits) has been carried out and the role

of each of them in electron transfer has been established (Schatz and Mason, 1974; Racker, 1975).

Along with the redox chain localised in the inner membrane and linked through the membrane potential to the mechanism' of conjugation, mitochondria have alternative pathways of electron transport (Skulachev, 1969), the components of which are represented in the outer membrane (Fig. 2). These redox systems bear different functional load and can be distinguished by selective respiratory poisons, for example, rotenone, which inhibits electron transport only along the respiratory chain of the inner mitochondrial membrane.

1.1. 2. **Structural and functional role of phospholipids of mitochondrial membranes.**

It should be noted that an essential point determining the normal functioning and interaction of mitochondrial enzyme systems is the intactness of the membrane structure, the main components of which are proteins and lipids. At the same time, phospholipids represent a component absolutely necessary for the normal course of the processes of energy transformation in the conjugation of the membrane.

Figure 2. Redox chain oxidation of NAD.H in the outer (rotenone-insensitive pathway) and inner (rotenone-sensitive pathway) mitochondrial membranes.

/The scheme is given according to V.P. Skulachev (1969)/.

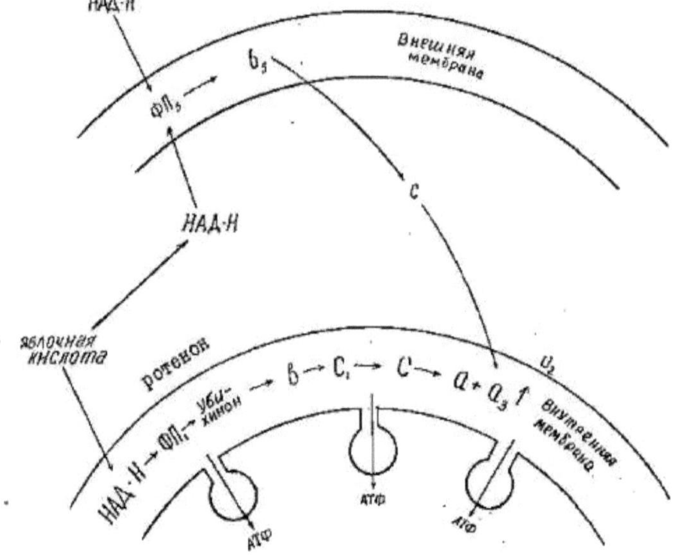

There is convincing evidence that phospholipids are not only a constituent part of membranes, they are required for virtually all membrane functions: oxidative phosphorylation (Crepe, 1981; Parenti- Casteilietal..., 1979; Pitottietal..., 1980), electron transfer (Pry, Green, 1981), transdehydrogenase (Rydstreemetal., 1975), and idehydrogenase (Rydstreemetal., 1975), 1979; Pitottietal., 1980), electron transfer (Pry, Green, 1981), transdehydrogenase (Rydstreemetal., 1975)idehydrogenase reactions (Vignais, 1976; Fleischeretal., 1977).

The main representatives of phospholipids are phosphoglycerides. The simplest representative of phosphoglycerides is phosphatidic acid. In biological membranes of mammalian cells phosphatidic acid is contained in insignificant amounts and is an intermediate product in the biosynthesis of other phosphoglycerides.

The most common phosphoglycerides in mammalian cells are phosphatidylcholine (PC), phosphatidylserine (PS), phosphatidyl ethanolamine (PE) and cardiolipin.

The major components of the phospholipid fraction of liver mitochondria are PC (39-44%), PE (25-37%) and cardiolipin (21-25%)

(Levyetal., I960; Stoffelet1980 1968; Mc-Murrayetal.,1972; Gazzotti, 1980).The phospholipid composition of liver, heart and kidney mitochondria has been found to be similar.

External and internal membranes also differ from each other in the content of individual phospholipid fractions (Levyetal., I960). The highest concentration of cardiolipin is most characteristic of the inner membranes of mitochondria, and of phosphatidylcholine of outer membranes. The amount of saturated fatty acids in phospholipids of outer membranes is higher than in inner membranes.

Intense incorporation of unsaturated fatty acids into the phospholipids of inner membranes was found by Keranen (1982).

Lipid-protein interactions in mitochondrial membranes are the most important factor in determining the functional state of organelles (Virjietal., 1978; Parenti-Castellietal., 1979). Phospholipids probably represent the "covering" material of mitochondrial enzyme complexes and play an important role in biological oxidation. It has been shown in a number of studies that the activity of many membrane enzymes is reduced or completely lost if phospholipids have been extracted from membranes. Removal of phospholipids from enzyme preparations depresses the activity of NAD.H- oxidase and NAD.H-cytochrome c-reductase (Fleischeretal,I977), kynurenine hydroxylase and monoamine oxidase (Kandasvamietal., 1978), rotenone-insensitive NAD.H-cytochrome-c-reductase (Feoetal., 1978), cytochrome oxidase (Fryetal., 1980).

Enzymatic activity is partially or completely restored by the addition of membrane phospholipids (Fleischeretal., 1977; Feoetal., 1978). Such enzymes include NAD.H-cytochrome-c reductase, cytochrome oxidase, NAD.H-oxidase, succinate-cytochrome-c reductase, glucose-6-phosphatase, and several others.

An analysis of the literature concerning the lipid dependence of enzyme activity leads to the conclusion that many enzymes require "common" lipid heads and certain types of fatty acids.

It should be noted, however, that local changes in the lipid microenvironment in invivoMoryT prove to be an important factor in metabolic control if the enzyme is membrane-bound.

According to some authors (Fleischer and Klouven, 1961; Brierleyetal., 1962; Szarkowska, 1966; lenazetal., 1971), removal of 70% or more of phospholipids causes complete inhibition of mitochondrial respiratory activity. This effect is reversible if the amount of phospholipids remaining in the preparation is at least 10%. Their further removal may lead to irreversible changes (Mikelsaar, Severina, Skulachev, 1974).

Not all lipids are equally effective in reactivating the mitochondrial respiratory chain. Both the type of phospholipid and its fatty acid composition are essential. It has also been observed that phospholipids of the same type, but obtained from different sources, are unequally active when reconstructed with mitochondrial systems devoid of phospholipids (Cabo-Soleretal, 1971).

Cytochrome oxidase has been found to contain a very tightly bound cardiolipin, which is removed only by the most rigid extraction (Awasthietal., 1970,1971; Chuangetal., I970; Hallman, Kankareetal.,I97I).Ha 1MOL OF enzyme contains 1MOL OF cardiolipin. The cleavage of firmly bound cardiolipin leads to the loss of cytochrome oxidase activity. It is restored only upon addition of cardiolipin (Chuangetal .,1970; Zanler , Fleischer, 1971).

Cytochrome oxidase preparations usually contain other phospholipids, but removal of 90% of this lipid material does not inactivate the enzyme. Preparations free of phosphatidylethanolamine and phosphatidylcholine, but containing cardiolipin, can be activated not by the addition of phospholipids but also fatty acids and even detergent. The degree of reactivation by individual phospholipids decreases in the following order: cardiolipin > mitochondrial phospholipid mixture> phosphatidylcholine > phosphatidylethanolamine, phosphatidylserine > phosphatidic acid. Phospholipids are thought to contribute to the proper interaction of cytochrome c with cytochrome oxidase (Thompson and Paks, 1972; Chuang and Crane, 1973).

Data of a different nature were obtained by studying cytochrome oxidase proteoliposomes prepared by dialysis.

When measuring proteoliposome respiration in the absence of dissociators of oxidative phosphorylation, phosphatidylcholine and phosphatidylethanolamine showed the same ability to activate the enzyme, and their mixture was slightly more effective. Cardiolipin was less active, with its addition reducing the activating effect of the other phospholipids. The picture changed dramatically when an uncoupler was introduced into the system; proteoliposomes containing cardiolipin oxidised ascorbate most intensively.

According to Bruni and Racker (Bruni and Racker, 1968), the activity of the electron transfer system at the cyKpHHaT-KoQ-pe,ayKTa3a stage does not depend on cardiolipin. Moreover, cardiolipin, starting at a certain concentration, prevents the activation of this system by a mixture of mitochondrial phospholipids. Egg phosphatidylcholine and phosphatidylethanolamine act weaker than a mixture of phospholipids from soya, the so-called azolectin, and do not activate succinate-KoQ reductase. Mitochondrial NAD.H-dehydrogenase (Lenazetal.,!971) reveals similar specificity with respect to phospholipids.

In a number of studies, the functions of phospholipids in electron transfer systems have been investigated using phospholipases A, C and D. Increasing the phospholipase concentration or longer incubation times cause almost complete inhibition of mitochondrial respiration. The process can be reactivated by the addition of certain phospholipids, the specificity of which is similar to that of preparations extracted with organic solvents (Machinist and Singer , 1965).

Bruni and Racker (1968) also studied succinate dehydrogenase, in the stabilisation and activity of which cardiolipin plays a special role. The authors note that other phospholipids contribute to the formation of the active complex of succinate dehydrogenase and cytochrome c, while cardiolipin is required for the activity of succinate dehydrogenase itself. NAD.H-dehydrogenase is the third component of the respiratory chain for which an important role of cardiolipin has been noted, at least in the structural organisation of this complex, since a direct correlation has been found between inhibition of enzyme activity and the amount of hydrolysed cardiolipin (Awasthietal., 1969). Cardiolipin is also attributed a specific structural and regulatory role in the functioning of glutamate dehydrogenase (Godinot, 1973).

As follows from the above, the interaction between phospholipids and proteins in the membrane is most important for the functional integrity of membrane-bound enzymes, including polyenzyme systems.

Phospholipids are able to maintain the optimal conformation of the catalytic centre of enzymes, and they are involved in the regulation of enzyme biosynthesis (Pitottietal., 1980; DiFrancescoetal., 1981). In the work of Augustinetal. (1977) it was shown that plasma membranes, mitochondria and post-mitochondrial fractions are involved in the synthesis of phospholipids. This process was found to be ATP-dependent.

I.I.3. **Structure and functions of mitochondria during embryogenesis.**

Tissue differentiation is characterised by an increase in the diversity of biochemical processes occurring in cells, which is accompanied by fluctuations in the functional activities of intracellular organelles. That is why mitochondria of differentiating tissues differ from mature mitochondria in structure and functions. Intensive growth of mitochondrial membranes occurs during embryonic development, differentiation of individual tissues and organs (Ozernyuk, 1978). Oocytes at the early stage of oogenesis contain mainly

small mitochondria with single cristae (Lamboni, Mastro-janni, 1966; Zybina, 1975).

Increases in mitochondrial size and cristae extension have been noted in early stages of embryonic development (Andersonetal., 1970; Baranaskaetal.,I976) and in later stages during growth and differentiation of tissues and organs (Weber, 1965; Mackieretal., 1971; ChedidetNair,I974).

On day 3 of development, mitochondria of chicken embryo liver parenchyma cells are few in number (a few mitochondria per cell) and have a filamentous structure. On day b mitochondria are already numerous and shorter in size. From this time until day 18 of development, they increase in size (Heisin, I960; Zagoruiko et al., 1975; Simonyan et al. 1977; StephansBils, 1967; Chedid, Nair, 1974. . In late embryonic development, elongated filamentous forms of mitochondria prevail, their density increases, and the structure of the cristae improves.

Before the birth of a rat or hatching of a chick, the number of elongated mitochondria decreases, rounded mitochondria, dumbbell-shaped and articulate forms appear, indicating the possibility of fragmentation of these organelles. The most noticeable changes occur in the embryonic and neonatal periods (Sentyurova, I975;Yeung, Oliver, 1968; Chuangetal., 1971).

In the mitochondria of the liver and brain of bird embryos, the systems of energy transformation are well developed (Simonyan, 1969; Makhinko and Shchegolkov, 1974). In mammalian embryos, this system becomes sufficiently perfect only in the postnatal period (Halimann, 197I; Nakazawaetal., 1973; Pollack, 1975).

During embryonic development, the contribution of cell organelles to the overall metabolism of the cell changes significantly. This may be a consequence of changes in the conditions inside the cell, as well as the process of self-maturation of cell organelles. Obviously, the changing functional load on mitochondria during embryogenesis is reflected in changes in both morphology and metabolism of liver mitochondria of mammals and birds (Khamidov et al., 1974; Besschetnikov, Chorayan, 1981; Dyatlovitskaya et al., 1982; Stephanes, Bils, 1967; Poliak, Woog, 1971; Duck-Chong, Poliak, 1973).

That is why mitochondria are the main supplier of ATP and some metabolites necessary for growth, development, organ differentiation and activity, detoxification, thermogenesis, etc.

During embryogenesis, not only the structure of mitochondria and the state of oxidative phosphorylation are modified, but also the activity of individual enzymes, metabolite and ion transport systems, etc. Thus, Poliak&Sutton(1980) showed that in fetal mitochondria (17-18 days) ATP is taken up faster than ADP and AMP is not accumulated. ATP is taken up against a concentration gradient, the rate of ATP accumulation is higher in fetal liver mitochondria than in adult animal liver mitochondria. $Mg+^2$ and $Ca+^2$ ions significantly increase and hexokinase inhibits ATP uptake by fetal rat liver mitochondria. $Mg+^2$, Ca^{+2} and hexokinase, according to the authors, may play a regulatory role in maintaining a low concentration of adenine nucleotides in fetal mitochondria and in the rapid increase in their content in mitochondria after rat birth.

It is interesting to note that the content of adenine nucleotides in the liver mitochondria of newborn rats increases several times between 2 and 3 hours after birth (Apriiie, 1981). When liver mitochondria of newborn rats are incubated with I mM ATP at 30° C for 10 minutes, the content of adenine nucleotides in liver mitochondria increases. Both the activity of adenine nucleotide translocase and the respiration rate of mitochondria in state 3 are increased. The mechanism of adenine nucleotide accumulation in newborn rat liver mitochondria is specific for ATP and ADP. The K values$_M$ for ATP and ADP at their capture by mitochondria are 0.857027 and 0.411020 mM, respectively, with ADP being a competitive inhibitor of ATP capture. Removal of inorganic phosphate from the incubation medium halved ATP and ADP capture by mitochondria. Mersalyl and N-ethylmaleimide inhibit the accumulation of adenine nucleotides in mitochondria. ATP uptake is stoichiometrically dependent on $MgCl_2$, indicating that magnesium ion is taken up by mitochondria along with ATP and ADP. The capture of ATP and especially ADP is stimulated by the addition of oxidisable substrates and inhibited by uncouplers of oxidative phosphorylation. Antimycin A has no effect on ATP capture but suppresses ADP capture. Carboxyatractyloside, in contrast, suppresses ATP uptake and has no effect on ADP capture. It is assumed that a specific adenine nucleotide transport system functions in the mitochondria of the liver of newborn rats, which is absent in adult animals.

Less studied is the ratio of oxidation and phosphorylation at different stages of embryogenesis and the role of free oxidation in differentiation processes.

Mitochondria isolated from intensively growing muscles of 18-day-old cockerels are characterised by a decrease in DC and P/0 values and a weak response to the action of respiration and phosphorylation uncouplers (Skulachev, 1962).

At the beginning of the fetal period, characterised by rapid growth, oxidation processes associated with phosphorylation prevail in the mitochondria of the liver and brain of chicken embryos and in the liver of duck embryos (Simonyan, 1969; Mahinko, Shchegolkov, 1974). Before hatching, the activity of oxidative phosphorylation decreases and ATPase activity increases. In the authors' opinion, these changes in energy metabolism reflect the peculiarities of growth and functioning of the liver during the foetal period.

It is known from the literature that the phospholipid composition of liver mitochondria changes significantly during chick embryogenesis (Koval, 1979; Dzhuraeva, 1983; Poolak and Woog, 1971). It has been shown that sphingomyelin and diphosphoinositide are absent in the brain homogenate or its subcellular fractions at early stages of rat or chick embryogenesis (Patrikeeva, 1964; Crepe, 1981). In the brain of the developing chicken embryo, they appear on day 16 of incubation, and their concentration increases with development. With increasing incubation period in mitochondria of heart and liver of chicken embryos and mitochondria of liver of rabbit embryos, the content of phospholipids increases (Zainutdinov et al., 1976; Dzhuraeva, 1983).

Bonini de Romanelli et al. (1981) studied the fatty acid composition and content of acidic phospholipids in subcellular fractions during the early development of the toad. It was found that the content of phosphatidic acid, phosphatidylserine, and phosphatidylinositol increased in the embryo at the gastrulation stage and especially in its mitochondrial fraction compared to unfertilised oocytes.

Thus, the change in the phospholipid composition of mitochondria during embryonic development is an undoubted fact and, apparently, contributes significantly to the corresponding state of the parameters of the functional state of mitochondria at different stages of embryogenesis.

1. 2. Effect of organophosphorus pesticides on physiological and biochemical processes of animal tissue cells.

Mass application of pesticides has led to their significant accumulation in the external environment and negative impact on many inhabitants of the biosphere, including humans and animals that are not direct objects of action of these compounds (Melnikov, 1973). An important point in terms of protecting the health of the population in contact with pesticides is the disclosure of the mechanisms of their action on human and animal organisms. This explains the necessity of versatile study of the mechanism of action of organophosphorus pesticides at various levels of structural organisation.

Entering the body of animals, organophosphorus pesticides are easily and rapidly absorbed, penetrating through the mucous membranes of the respiratory tract, gastrointestinal tract, eyes and skin, possess a narrow zone of toxic action and the ability to both functional (Kagan, 1970; Kundiev, 1975) and material cumulation (Bear, 1977).

Signs of poisoning for most organophosphorus compounds are largely similar, since the leading mechanism of action of these compounds is inhibition of cholinesterase activity, i.e. influence on cholinergic synapses. However, along with this main mechanism, organophosphorus pesticides cause a variety of disturbances in most other physiological functions, biochemical processes, and the structure of cells and subcellular organelles.

Thus, when chlorophos was administered to animals at a dose of I/100 LD_{50} (daily, orally), the activity of alanine and aspartate trans-ferase, alkaline phosphatase and cholinesterase of the liver did not differ significantly from the control, but cellular elements without nucleus were found in small numbers.

After 6 months, the dyscomplementation becomes more permanent, hepatocytes with polyploid nuclei are found, small fatty dystrophy is noted, the amount of glycogen and RNA is reduced. After 8 months, the discomplexity becomes significant, there are more nucleusless cells, the number of cell elements with polyploid nuclei and small hepatocytes increases (Rodionov and Voronina, 1973).

The function of higher nervous activity is disturbed under the action of low doses of phosphamide (Panshina, 1963). Reactivity of blood cholinesterase decreases already after I hour in blood serum by 39-59%, in erythrocytes by 58-82%. When the concentration of pesticide decreases, the depressing effect on cholinesterase decreases accordingly.

Decrease in cholinesterase activity was observed under the influence of most organophosphorus pesticides: methaphos (Trefilov, Faerman, 1965), chlorophos (Tsapko, 1965), phthalophos (Knysh, 1980), methylnitrophos and DDVF (Kagan et al. 1970) and others. Prolonged administration of various doses of butifos (1/50, 1/20

LD_{50}) leads to a sharp decrease in the activity of intestinal monoglyceridlipase (Zakirov et al., 1975; Kadirov et al., 1982). Even a small dose of the preparation (1/50LD_{50}) already on the 15th day of inoculation resulted in almost threefold decrease of the activity of this enzyme. By the end of the first month it remained at the same level, and from the 60th day there was a tendency to its recovery. On the 15th and 30th day of the experiment the activity of cholinesterase in blood sharply decreased.

When butifos is administered within 6 days at a dose of 1/50 LD_{50} , the drug causes in the liver dilation of portal tract vessels, central veins, leads to accumulation of glycogen, dystrophic changes in epithelial cells with a decrease in their RNA content (Nadzhimutdinov et al., 1975). Butifos administration during 4 months at a dose of 4.1 mg/kg body weight decreased liver protein content and increased lipid content. Morphological changes in the liver were reduced to signs of moderate circulatory disorders and dystrophic changes of epithelial cells; a decrease in RNA and glycogen content was also found (Knyazeva et al. 1974). Administration of this pesticide for 10 months at a dose of 1/20 LD_{50} had practically no effect on the content of proteins and glycogen in the liver (Khakimov et al., 1973), whereas the content of total lipids increased.

When butifos was administered at a dose of 1/20LD_{50} for I month, the activity of monoglyceridlipase, glycylvalindipeptidase, invertase, amylase in the small intestine decreased. After a six-day administration of this pesticide, a slight increase in protein and total lipids was noted in the liver. With repeated and prolonged administration, there was a significant fluctuation in glycogen content, both decreasing and increasing. After 6-day and 4-month administration of butifos, the decrease in the level ofproteins was significant (Hakimov et al., 1973). Judging by the literature data, no significant increase in the noted shifts is observed during long-term administration of butifos in the future. Apparently, under conditions of chronic intoxication of the organism, liver cells undergo certain compensatory changes, which allow preserving functional activity of hepatocytes for a long time.

Daily administration of methylmercaptophos to rabbits at a dose of I mg/kg of weight causes changes in morphological composition of blood and activity of serum transaminases in experimental animals. No special changes were observed in total protein. Throughout the experiment, the content of globulins was increased and albumin decreased (Kur et al., 1973).

When one of the representatives of organophosphorus pesticides, phosphamide, was administered on day 10, no pronounced shifts in the ratio of protein fractions were observed, while on day 20 there was an increase in the content of -globulins and insignificant increase in the level of - and -globulins. On day 30, changes in the protein composition of blood serum were very pronounced and were characterised by significant hy- poalbuminemia and hyperglobulinemia mainly due to - and - globulins (Jamalutdinov, 1974).

According to Akhmerova (1970), exposure to low doses of pesticides does not cause clinical manifestations of poisoning. However, in the organism of experimental animals there is a defensive-adaptive, compensatory reaction, and in case of long-term experiments - morphological changes. At low doses the changes were non-specific and reversible.

Under the influence of phosphamide and chlorophos of low intensity in peripheral blood its indices change. Akhmadjanov (1976) found that the activity of alkaline phosphatase, peroxidase, as well as the amount of phospholipids and glycogen decreases under the influence of these pesticides.

When antio is administered at a dose of I/I00 LD_{50} , a gradual decrease in cholinesterase activity is observed, which reaches a maximum by day 70 of inoculation. With increasing duration of antio exposure, suppression of adrenal cortex hormone secretion occurs (Kurambaev, 1981). Phthalophos also caused pronounced changes in the liver in the form of an increase in the number of dinuclear parenchyma cells, appearance of mitosis figures, proliferation of kupffer cells, and polyploidy of hepatocyte nuclei (Rodionov, 1974). Akhmerova et al. (1976) noted that during intragastric administration of small doses of butifos there were observed dystrophic and inflammatory processes in the liver, decrease of RNA and sharp fatty degeneration of hepatocytes, which is, according to the authors, the result of hypoxia and violation of oxidative processes.

After aerosol treatment of sheep with phthalophos at a dose of 100 mg per kg of weight, some decrease or deviation from normal distribution of glycogen in the liver and heart, increase in succinate dehydrogenase activity were observed. However, deviations in the content of glycogen, cholinesterase, succinate dehydrogenase were short-lived and did not cause visible clinical disorders in the organism (Knysh, 1980). Under the influence of phthalophos, the nucleic acid content in the gonads is reduced. Reduction of the administered dose to 1/300LD_{50} was accompanied by shifts similar to those observed during the action of 1/100LD_{50} (Anina, 1975).

In the pathogenesis of poisoning by organophosphorus compounds, besides specific inhibition of cholinesterase, apparently, there may be other non-specific mechanisms of their action, which have been little studied so far. Organochlorine pesticides have been shown to have the ability to damage chromosomes, resulting in irreversible mutations. No such data are available for organophosphorus pesticides. However, it is known that a single administration of a toxic dose of chlorophos (500 mg/kg) to rats causes changes in the content of nucleic acids in liver tissue, especially nuclear nucleic acids. The observed changes have a phase character: in the first day their quantity decreases, and from 3 days their increase begins, which is maintained during the subsequent period of observations (up to 20 days). The increase in the amount of nuclear nucleic acids in liver tissue and the content of nucleic acids in terms of I g of dry weight of nuclei on the 1st day after exposure to chlorophos is characteristic for processes of liver destruction. The changes observed on the 3rd day after inoculation are characteristic for the processes of liver regeneration. In distant terms compensatory reactions of regulation of synthesis and decay of nucleic acids, as well as cell division, leading to normalisation of biochemical functions of the organism (Toropova, Egorova, 1967).

Administration of methylnitrophos and DDVF at a dose of $1/20LD_{50}$ caused a pronounced change in carbohydrate metabolism. In particular, a decrease in glycogen content and an increase in the amount of pyruvic acid in blood were observed (Kagan et al., 1970). The ratio of protein fractions of blood serum in rats was characterised by a sharp decrease in albumin content and increase in globulin fractions,

especially and Significant changes in the proteinogram, observed one month after the beginning of the experiment, gradually normalised by the 6th month. The same authors showed that protein-synthetic and excretory function of the liver was the most sensitive to the effect of DDVF.

Thus, analysis of the literature data indicates that different organophosphorus pesticides studied under similar experimental conditions cause similar histomorphological and functional changes.

1. 3 Effects of pesticides on structure and function mitochondria.

There is a number of contradictory data on the effect of organophosphorus pesticides on tissue respiration in the literature. Zhdanovich and Udalov (1969) observed an increase in succinate dehydrogenase activity in brain, kidney and heart tissues with simultaneous inhibition of cytochrome oxidase activity when animals were poisoned with subtoxic doses of dipterex. Kovalenok and Casanova (1967) found a decrease in succinate dehydrogenase activity in the tissues of insects poisoned with chlorophos. Zabusov (1967), however, found no change in the activity of succinate dehydrogenase and cytochrome oxidase in FOS-poisoned animals. Karmilov (1974) found, on the other hand, that administration of chlorophos at a dose of 300 mg/kg to rats for 5 days depressed the activity of succinate dehydrogenase and cytochrome oxidase of brain tissue and internal organs. More pronounced suppression of succinate dehydrogenase activity than cytochrome oxidase was noted. At the same time, studies by Gulyamov et al, (1981) showed that administration of chlorophos at a dose of 1/20 LD_{50} for 15 days increases the respiration rate of liver mitochondria in the resting state, while phosphorylating - decreases, resulting in a decrease in the value of respiratory control. At 75 days of chlorophos inoculation, oxygen consumption by mitochondria in active metabolic states proceeded at approximately the same rate as at 15 days of administration. However, the respiratory control coefficient was increased at the same time due to a significant decrease in the respiration rate of mitochondria in the resting state. The efficiency of oxidative phosphorylation when succinate was oxidised had a greater tendency to normalise, compared with glutamate as an oxidation substrate.

Studies by Dolgo-Saburov et al. (1982) showed that 4 hours after intramuscular administration of chlorophos to female rats at a dose of 300 mg/kg, the content of mitochondrial membrane phospholipids increased. The change in phospholipid content, according to these researchers, is considered to be the result of inhibition of their metabolism. No changes in phospholipid biosynthesis were found under the action of chlorophos.

When animals are exposed to chlorophos, the activity of oxidase systems of the respiratory chain of liver mitochondria does not change significantly (Gulyamov et al., 1981). However, more significant changes in the activity of the studied'polyenzyme systems (NAD.H-oxidase, succinatoxidase and cytochrome c-oxidase) of liver mitochondria of animals exposed to chlorophos were observed during thermal degradation of mitochondria, as well as during the action of controlled amounts of phospholipase A_2 or trypsin. At the same time, mitochondria from experimental rats showed faster inactivation of the above mentioned polyenzyme systems, which, in the authors' opinion, is associated with the presence of "hidden" disorders of structural relationships between proteins and phospholipids in the composition of mitochondrial membranes.

When studying the effect of chlorophos at a dose of 1/20 LD_{50} on respiration, oxidative phosphorylation and activity of polyenzyme systems of mitochondria of rat pancreas under shuAo conditions, it was found that during 15 days there is a suppression of respiration and efficiency of ATP synthesis (Almatov and Gulyamov, 1981). However, on the 75th day of the experiment the indices of oxidative phosphorylation normalise to some extent, although the rate of substrate oxidation remains reduced.

In bazudine poisoning, disorders of carbohydrate, lipid metabolism (Khalikov et al., 1981) and oxidative phosphori-

liver mitochondria (Saidkasymova et al., 1981; Khalikov et al., 1981). Disruption of the activity of membrane-bound enzymes of the respiratory chain and "incorporation" of exogenous cytochrome into the inner membrane of mitochondria have also been observed (Khalikov et al., 1981).

Studies by Hakimov et al. (1975) showed that as a result of a single injection of butifos at a dose of 1/50 LD_{50} the activity of ATPase and cytochrome oxidase increased, and the activity of succinate dehydrogenase decreased. After 6 days, the activity of all investigated enzymes decreased. By the end of the month period, a tendency to normalisation was observed in the activity of the studied enzymes. The same authors noted that during acute intoxication with butifos at a dose of 1/3 LD_{50} the activity of cytochrome oxidase and Mg^{2+} -ATPase slightly increased, and the activity of succinate dehydrogenase decreased. A decrease in the activity of the latter enzyme is also observed when antio is administered at a dose of 1/20 LDzd after 20 days from the start of administration (Sologub et al., 1974). However, in subsequent periods an increase is noted. Butifos does not depress the activity of succinate dehydrogenase throughout the experiment, even during the recovery period. Decrease in succinate dehydrogenase activity during exposure to chlorophos at a concentration of 61 mg/m^3 for 6 months was also noted by Knysh (1980), as well as during the use of pesticide BI-58 at a concentration of 0.05 mg/m^3 (Kaloyanova et al., 1968). Karmilov (1973,1974), studying the effect of chlorophos at a dose of 300 mg/kg, found a decrease in the activity of succinate dehydrogenase and cytochrome oxidase in the

liver, heart and kidneys.
When studying the functional activity of mitochondrial particles under the influence of phthalophos, chlorophos and herbicides - atrozine and dimetrine, it was found that the studied pesticides are inhibitors of NAD..H-oxidase, and their inhibitory activity depends on the nature and concentration of the substances used (Shabarchin et al., 1977).
When studying the effect of butifos at a dose of $1/50LD_{50}$ for I and 6 days, I, 2, 4 and 10 months with daily administration, it was found that in all variants of the experiment butifos increases the value of DA, while the value of ADP/0 does not differ significantly from the control (Khakimov et al., 1975). During acute intoxication at a dose of 1/3 LD_{50} , 24 hours after the administration of butifos. significantly increases respiration in V_4 h V_3 , *but* insignificantly decreases the rate of oxygen consumption in V_4 . These changes result in an increase in the magnitude of DA. It is known that a decrease in respiration rate in the controlled state (V_4) indicates increased energy regulation, while an increase in the value of DA indicates increased mitochondrial coupling. From this we can conclude that as a result of butyphos administration the liver mitochondria (strange as it may seem!) are in an optimally energised state (Khakimov et al., 1975). Based on the above, it can be assumed that the energy supply of hepatocytes during butyphos administration is in a satisfactory state.
When studying the effect of antio and methylmercaptophos at a dose of $1/20LD_{50}$ AND butiphos at a dose of $1/20LD_{50}$ when administered daily for 40 days, it was found that the energy level of liver mitochondria significantly decreases 2 months after the beginning of the experiment. By the end of the recovery period the indices of respiration and oxidative phosphorylation of liver mitochondria of experimental rats become close to the control ones (Kur, 1974).
Skoniecznaetal. (1981) investigated the respiratory activity of
of rat brain mitochondria of different ages under the action of chlorfenvinphos and found that this drug reduces the rate of oxygen consumption by mitochondria in the V3 state, the inhibition deepens with increasing concentration of the drug and with the age of these animals.
Olorunsogoetal. (1979) showed that 5 hours after intraperitoneal administration of the herbicide compound \'-(phos-fomethyl)-glycine to rats, a marked inhibition of energy-dependent phosphate-induced swelling of isolated liver mitochondria was observed. Administration of 60, 120 and 240 mg of this drug per I kg of rat live weight resulted in inhibition of mitochondrial swelling by 20, 40 and 65%, respectively, for both oxidation-oxybutyrate and succinate. The authors believe that this action of this drug is due to the fact that it is an uncoupler of oxidative phosphorylation. Indeed, N-phosphomethylglycine at a concentration of $6.25.10^{-4}$ M increases approximately 2-fold the rate of oxidation of succinate and -oxybutyrate in the absence of ADP (Bababunmietal., 1979). Respiratory control is reduced and simultaneously ATPase activity of liver mitochondria is increased. This pesticide relieves the inhibition of oxidation induced by oligomycin. The authors conclude that this organophosphorus

compound exhibits the properties of a dinitrophenol-type disassembler.
Sitkewiezetal. (1975,1976) investigated the activity of cyto-chromo-s oxidase and succinate dehydrogenase in rat brain mitochondria at different times after ingestion of dipterex and dichlofos at doses of 2-10-50 LD_{50} . The authors found that dipterex had no appreciable effect. Decrease in cytochrome c oxidase activity was observed after single or multiple administration of large doses of dichlofos to animals, but no changes in succinate dehydrogenase activity were observed.
After 10-day intraperitoneal administration of parathion (I mg/kg body weight) to rats, the respiration of liver mitochondria was also reduced if the oxidation substrate was a mixture of glutamate+malate+malonate, but the inhibitory effect of this drug was not observed with succinate (Spetaleetal.,1977). The authors suggest that parathion is an inhibitor of the electron transport system via the NAD-dependent pathway of the mitochondrial respiratory chain, i.e. it has an amytal-like action.
Shabarchin et al. (1977, 1979) studied the effect of chlorophos, metaphos, phthalophos, promethrin, strasin and desmethrin on the NAD.H-oxidase activity of submitochondrial particles from bovine heart. The authors found that the mentioned pesticides are inhibitors of NAD.H-oxidase and their effectiveness increases with increasing concentration. Other researchers have found that chlorfenvinphos and its analogues inhibit the oxygen consumption state in rat brain mitochondria, with chlorfenvinphos acting most strongly (Sitkewiczetal., 1978). However, at concentrations of 25- 75 μM these compounds do not affect the respiration rate of mitochondria in the state (succinate is the substrate of oxidation), nor does the activity of succinate dehydrogenase and cytochrome c-oxidase change.
An inhibitory effect of trichlorophene on the activity of cytochrome-c-oxidase after incubation with dissociated mitochondria was found under in vitro conditions (Sitkewicz and Zolewska, 1975; Sitkewiczetal., 1976). However, when intact mitochondria were incubated with trichlorophene, no changes in cyt-chloro-e oxidase activity were observed. Dichlorophos in both solubilised and intact mitochondria fractions caused stimulation of cytochrome oxidase activity. Both pesticides had no effect on succinate dehydrogenase activity.
Spetaleetal. (1977) studied the effect of organophosphorus pesticides parathion, malathion and dimethoate on the respiration of rat liver mitochondria. It was shown that the drugs used in concentrations above 26 μg/ml significantly inhibited the respiration rate of mitochondria in the presence of 2,4-DNF. It is interesting to note that a similar effect was observed without the addition of the uncoupler.
Thus, the analysis of literature data allows us to consider that in the pathogenesis of organophosphorus pesticide poisoning a significant role belongs to oxidative and bioenergetic processes disorders. The effects of pesticides on energy and oxidative metabolism of animal tissue cells largely depend on the structure of a particular preparation, the dose used, the terms of administration and a number of other conditions. It is essential to emphasise that in most cases oxidation of NAD-dependent substrates is subjected to

to the influence of pesticides to a greater extent than succinate oxidation. Under the influence of the introduction of FOS preparations in the mitochondrial population such disturbances in the functioning of oxidase systems are formed, which can be detected by the inactivation kinetics under the action of temperature or lytic enzymes. The above-mentioned material also unambiguously testifies that under the influence of pesticides of phosphorus-organic nature significant rearrangements occur in the structure and metabolism of tissues, cells and subcellular formations. In other words, pesticides of this type are not only cholinesterase inhibitors, but also non-specific structural and metabolic poisons. Their embryotoxic and teratogenic effects are also well known, which will be discussed briefly in the next section.

1. 4. Effect of pesticides on embryo growth and development.

The effect of chlorophos on embryogenesis of warm-blooded animals was studied by a number of researchers at different routes of pesticide ingestion.

Hofmekler and Tabakova (1970) studied the effect of chlorophos at concentrations of 0.2, 0.02 and 0.055 mg/m^3 at continuous inhalation intake into the rat organism during the whole gestation period (20 days). It was found that all investigated concentrations had a distinct embryotropic effect, manifested by the presence of external and internal abnormalities of embryo development - incomplete ossification of the spine and the end of the ribs in embryos, the appearance of extra bones in the lower limbs. Weight indicators of organs and embryo change, there are deviations in the content of ascorbic and nucleic acids in the tissues of the female and foetus, the presence of histopathological and histochemical changes in the placenta.

The effect of chlorophos on the embryogenesis of rats by peros administration is less pronounced than by inhalation. Thus, after administration of chlorophos at a dose of 8 mg/kg throughout the entire gestation period, only a few cases of wavy curved vertebrae were observed (Marfsonetal., 1976).

When chlorophos was fed to rats with food at doses of 145, 375,432 mg/kg daily, fetuses showed developmental anomalies, the frequency of which increased with increasing chlorophos dose. Decrease in daily feed consumption and weight gain, death of some animals at intragastric administration of pesticide were observed. Chlorophos caused a decrease in body weight of offspring, morphological changes in the skeleton, but did not increase mortality compared to the control (Staples et al., 1975; Staplesetal., 1976).

A single injection of chlorophos into the stomach at a dose of 80 mg/kg on the 13th day of gestation caused an increase in post-implantation fetal death in rats. The following abnormalities were observed in living foetuses: exencephaly, hydrocephaly, and the symptom of "eyelids not closing" (Martson et al., 1975). The authors, however, believe that in this case the em-briotoxic and teratogenic effects of chlorophos are manifested at doses much higher than the actual amount of the drug that can enter the human body, and therefore it does not pose a practically teratogenic danger to humans when administered orally.

Leibovich (1973) studied the effect of low doses of chlorophos and methaphos on offspring obtained from hunted animals. It was found that the combined oral administration of chlorophos and methaphos showed more pronounced embryotokic effects of the pesticides than their isolated effects. Pesticides at a dose of 0.1 mg/kg and higher affected the generative function of animals, caused a decrease in their ability to conceive and reduced fertility.

The presence of selective embryotoxic and teratogenic phthalophos has been reported by many investigators (Voronina, 1971; Kagan, 1972; Marfsonetal., 1976),

When phthalophos was administered at a dose of 0.3 mg/kg (administered every other day throughout pregnancy), single foetuses with external deformities (trunk oedema, hind limb dislocation, pelvic girdle overstretching, jaw bone disorder) were found. Examination of the state of internal organs revealed various malformations (hydrocephalus, gerorrhagia, etc.). The rats of experimental females had lower weight and cranio-caudal dimensions in comparison' with the control ones. The experiments showed that in doses of 15, 7.5, 1.5 and 0.3 mg/kg phthalophos negatively affects the intrauterine development of the foetus, and in the dose of 0.06 mg/kg it does not affect the studied parameters.

Kasymova (1975) studied the embryotoxic effect of butifos at a single intragastric administration of its various doses to rats in different periods of pregnancy. It was found that butifos in doses of 24.5 and 12.5 mg/kg caused high, statistically significant mortality of foetuses, reduction of their weight and cranio-caudal dimensions. Hofmekler (1974), studying the effects of butifos at average daily MAC throughout pregnancy, found embryotoxic and teratogenic effects of butifos.

Budreu&Singh (1973) in experiments on CF-1 mice established embryotoxic and teratogenic properties of mercaptophos and fenthion. The authors believe that the teratogenic effect of these organophosphorus pesticides is not related to their cholinesterase properties.

Khuriev et al. (1969), Hofmekler (1971; 1974) studied the properties of methylmercaptophos on embryogenesis of rats at 24-hour inhalation intake in different concentrations. As a result of the study it was determined that under the influence of methylmercaptophos at concentrations of 0.0003, 0.1 and 0.5 mg/m^3 embryo death was sharply increased. Post-implantation fetal mortality, although increasing with increasing pesticide concentration, did not increase significantly (Hofmekler et al., 1969).

The effect of methylmercaptophos on embryogenesis was also studied by other routes of pesticide administration. Thus, Sayramanova (1971) studied the effect of methylmercaptophos on embryogenesis of white rats when administered orally for 10 days, starting from the 5th or 10th day of pregnancy. Embryo death was noted in females that received the drug in both the first and second half of pregnancy. Similar data were obtained when methylmercaptophos was administered to the stomach of white rats on the 9th and 13th days of pregnancy (Levskaya, 1973).

Introduction of thiophos into chicken yolk in doses of 0.25 - I mg at different stages of embryogenesis caused abnormalities of skeletal development in chicken embryos

(Lutz-Osiertoyetal., 1969). Abnormal development of the axial skeleton in embryos was observed in the form of fusion of vertebral arches at the action of the drug on the 4th and 10th day of incubation. Disturbance of the structure of other organs was also noted.

Proctoretal. (1975) studied the effect of a number of organophosphorus insecticides on the NAD content of chicken embryos. Insecticides were sterile injected into the yolk sac of fertilised chicken eggs on day 4 of incubation. On day 12, NAD was determined in eggs, and on day 18, embryos were examined for gross anatomical deformities. There was an inverse correlation between the incidence, severity of deformities and NAD levels. Nicotinamide administration eliminated or significantly attenuated the teratogenic effect of organophosphorus insecticides.

The use of chicken embryos as experimental models makes it possible to trace the initial reaction of the embryo to the direct introduction of a pesticide. Foreign chemicals, when introduced into the chicken egg, persist in the egg for a long time and thus have a damaging effect on embryonic cells. In mammals, before an exogenous chemical can affect embryonic cells, it must pass through the germinal membranes, or placental barrier, where enzyme systems function to break down or selectively accumulate xenobiotics. Therefore, the positive results of the experiment on chicken embryos indicate the feasibility of conducting similar studies using other animal species.

Pish (1966) revealed the embryotoxic effect of thiophos in experiments on rats. When this drug was administered from day 7 to 15 of pregnancy, high postnatal mortality was observed. Fetuses showed subcutaneous haematomas, depressed cholinesterase activity in the brain, and decreased body weight. Kimbrough (1968) found embryotoxic properties of this insecticide at doses that did not cause intoxication in pregnant rats, i.e. in these experiments the selective effect of thiophos on the embryo organism was revealed.

It was found that administration of chlorfenvinphos to chicken embryos on the 6th or 10th day of incubation at concentrations of 0.125 and 0.5 mg, regardless of the time of administration, caused death of embryos with increasing concentration of the pesticide. When the same drug was administered to pregnant rats, osteogenesis was disturbed in foetuses, while no changes were observed in organs of females (Tos-Lutyetal., 1972).

Dichlofos, a contact insecticide widely used, when administered to rabbits at a dose of 6 mg/kg for 10 days before parturition, decreased cholinesterase activity in fetal brain homogenates (Masiinskaetal., 1978). Changes were also observed in Broca's nuclei, olfactory medulla, and in the nuclei of the optic tubercle.

When rats were administered Valexon and chlorophos at doses of 1/20 and 1/100 LD_{50} daily throughout pregnancy or during critical periods of offspring development, it was found that pesticides create conditions for the emergence of "chemical stress", the expression of which is the disruption of neuro-humoral regulation, the development of a state of "activation-exhaustion" in the mother-fetus system (Badaeva et al., 1981).

Laleyetal. (1977) studied the effect of carbophos. The authors noted hypoglycaemia in fetuses due to increased differentiation of islets of Langerhans, and a direct correlation was observed between the severity of micromyelia in fetuses and hypoglycaemia. Leibovich (1973) and Kimbrough (1968), studying the effect of carbophos on rat embryogenesis, did not reveal either embryotoxic or teratogenic properties of the drug. Disruption of embryonic development depends largely on the ability of chemicals to pass the placental barrier.

Pish (1966), when studying the activity of cholinesterase in the brain of embryos after the introduction of organophosphorus pesticides - thiophos, methaphos and DDF - found a suppression of the activity of this enzyme, which indicates the permeability of the placenta to pesticides. This is also evidenced by the data of Ackemann(1974), who after the introduction of pregnant rats methaphos, bromophos and phthalophos established after 30 minutes the presence of pesticides in the placenta, liver, brain and muscle tissues of the foetus, Budreauetal. (1973) investigated the transplacental transfer of mercaptophos. Mass radioactivity was noted in the placenta 20 minutes after administration to SR mice and decreased after 2 hours. Among the examined fetal tissues, the highest radioactivity was observed in osteogenic mesenchyme. This suggests that mercaptophos is absorbed by the tissues of the maternal organism and rapidly penetrates through the placenta. Staszycetal. (1974) believe that chlorophos when administered to pregnant rats penetrates through the placenta and has a cytotoxic effect on the fetal cell. Transplacental transfer of pesticides thiophos, metaphos, DDVF, TEPF is evidenced by studies of Hathwoyetal. (1972) and Kimbroughetal. (1968). A similar conclusion was obtained when studying the distribution of phthalophos in the organism of pregnant rats and foetus (Voronina, 1971).

During pregnancy, physiological changes occur in the body to preserve the embryo and its further development. The combination of changes in the maternal body may have a multifaceted effect on the metabolism of chemical compounds that have entered it from the environment, and may be accompanied by some slowing of metabolism and prolonged excretion of metabolites and the drugs themselves from the pregnant woman's body. The metabolism of chemicals in the pregnant woman is closely linked to the functioning of the foetoplacental system.

The placenta consists of actively metabolising tissue, significantly modifies metabolic processes in the body and forms a complex barrier between the maternal and foetal circulatory systems. Substances that have a damaging effect on the development of the embryo can manifest their pathogenic effect by penetrating the placenta.

Since most of the preparations are fat-soluble substances, it is natural that they accumulate in the lipid layer of biomembranes and, in particular, in mitochondrial membranes, having a non-specific effect on their permeability, respiration and energy transformation processes. In this connection it is of undoubted interest to study the effect of pesticides on the energy metabolism of the liver of embryos, pregnant rabbits and placenta. It is noted that in the mechanism of toxic effect of organophosphorus compounds along with anticholinesterase effect an important role belongs to the disturbance of the function of energy-transforming systems of the cell (Shabarchin et al., 1977; Abo-Khatwaa.Hollingworth, 1974; Spetoleetal., 1977).

When chlorophos was administered daily to rabbits at doses of 50 and 75 mg/kg starting from the 2nd day of pregnancy, chlorophos did not cause disturbances in the course of pregnancy (haemorrhage, miscarriages) and developmental anomalies noticeable to the naked eye, but reduced respiration of placenta tissues and fetal organs (Andrashko et al., 1975). The maximum effect was observed in the placenta on day 15-16 of gestation under the influence of 75 mg chlorophos/kg. On day 29-30 of gestation, the greatest decrease in the intensity of oxygen uptake occurred in the liver of the foetus. The decrease in the intensity of tissue respiration was deepened by increasing the dose of the drug while decreasing the period of its exposure to the pregnant female. A similar picture was obtained in studies by Campo (1982,1983): chlorophos, without interrupting the course of pregnancy, has a significant effect on metabolism in the placenta.

The results of the study of the electron-transport chain of mitochondria of the placenta of rabbits poisoned with chlorophos (on the 27-29th day of gestation, at a dose of 175 mg/kg), using different oxidation substrates, indicate a dissociation of the oxidation and phosphorylation process at the cytochrome section of the respiratory chain (Akberov, 1978).

As evidenced by literature data, the possibility of adverse effect of pesticides on embryogenesis has been investigated mainly from the classical positions of evaluation of certain anomalies: fecundity, intrauterine death, developmental deformities, weight indices of embryos and their organs, placenta, pathomorphological, separate biochemical studies of female and embryo organs. These studies make it possible to characterise the degree of disturbance, but they are not sufficient to reveal the mechanism of various disorders of metabolic processes caused by pesticides. To solve such problems it seems necessary to study the functional state of cells and subcellular organelles, in particular, oxidative phosphorylation, activity of some membrane-bound organelles, as well as the activity of pesticide-induced metabolic processes.

mitochondrial enzymes, changes in phospholipid and protein fractions of mitochondrial membranes of various maternal and foetal organs. That is why we studied respiration and oxidative phosphorylation, activity of NAD.H-oxidase, succinatoxidase and cy-tochrome c-oxidase, as well as phospholipid and protein composition of maternal and fetal liver mitochondrial membranes under the action of one of the representatives of organophosphorus pesticides - butifos, widely used in cotton growing as a defoliant.

EXPERIMENTAL PART

Chapter 2

Materials and Methods.

2. 1.Object of the study.

Ingestion of animals with butifos was performed on days 13 and 19 of rabbit gestation intragastrically using a special probe. The dose of butifos was 1/20 LD_{50} . Experiments were conducted in winter and autumn, animals were slaughtered 10 days after inoculation.

Embryonic liver, placenta and maternal liver were used for mitochondria isolation.

2.2. A method for isolating mitochondria.

Mitochondria from the liver of embryos, maternal organism and placenta were isolated using the common method of differential centrifugation proposed by Schneider, Hogeboom (1950), Parsons, Simson (1967). Mitochondria from placenta, foetuses were isolated according to the method of Swirczynskietal(1976). Rabbits were decapitated, liver was extracted and placed in a beaker with chilled medium of the following composition: sucrose 250 mM, Tris 20 mM, EDTA 20 mM, pH = 0.5 mM.
7.4. After determining the liver weight, the liver pieces were crushed using a press with a stainless steel filter (hole diameter 0.8 mm). The resulting pulp was homogenised in a glass homogeniser with a Teflon pestle with 8-10 times the volume of cold extraction medium. Nuclei and cell fragments were removed by centrifugation at 600 g for 15 min at 0-2 °C. Mitochondria were precipitated at 8000g for 15 min. The resulting mitochondria were resuspended in the extraction medium and centrifuged again at 750 g to purify them from blood elements.

The placenta was washed in 0.9% NaCl solution, then in 0.25 mM sucrose containing 5 mM EDTA, 10 mM Tris-HCl1, pH = 7.4, after which the tissue was crushed with a press, homogenised and filtered through three-layer gauze. The placenta homogenate was centrifuged at 2300 for I min. The supernatant was centrifuged at 16000g for 3 min. The resulting mitochondria were resuspended in the extraction medium but without EDTA, then centrifuged at 500g for 5 min. The supernatant was centrifuged again at 7000g for 10 min. Mitochondria were resuspended in a solution containing 0.25 mM sucrose, 10 mM Tris, pH = 7.4.

2.3. Determination of mitochondrial respiration and oxidative phosphorylation.

The rate of oxygen consumption by mitochondria was measured by polarographic method on a PPT-I polarograph; using a rotating platinum electrode under standard conditions at 25 °C. The ADP/0 and DA ratios were expressed according to Chance-Williams. The incubation medium used for liver mitochondria from embryos and pregnant rabbits was KCI 120 mM, KH_2 $P0_4$ 5 mM, Tris 10 mM, pH=7.4. For placental mitochondria, the medium used was: KCI 15 mM, Tris 50 mM, KH_2 RO_4 20 mM, $MgSO_4$ 5 mM, EDTA 2 mM, cytochrome c 10 μM, bovine albumin 0.5%. Succinate and glutamate were used as oxidation substrate.

2. 4 Determination of the activity of polyenzyme systems of mitochondrial membranes.

NAD. H-oxidase and succinatoxidase activities of mitochondria were determined according to the method of Hatefietal. (1962) as modified by Rakhimov and Almatov (1977). Rotenone-insensitive and rotenone-sensitive NAD. H-oxidase activity was determined according to the method of Ernsteretal. (1963), cytochrome-c-oxidase activity was determined according to the method of Wharton and Griffiths (1961). Mitochondria subjected to a single freeze-thaw treatment were used in the experiment. The measurement medium contained 0.66 M sucrose, 5 mM histidine, 50 mM Tris-HCl, pH = 7.4. The following amounts of substrates were used to measure enzyme activity. The final concentration of substrates in the cell was: NAD.H - I mM, succinate - 10 mM, ascorbate - 20 mM, cytochrome c - 0.4 mg/ml. Rotenone was used in an amount of 2 µmol/ml. Enzymatic activities were expressed in µmols of oxygen consumed per I min per I mg of mitochondrial protein.

2. 5 Determination of phospholipid content.

Lipid extraction was performed according to the Folchetal method (Folchetal., 1957). Mitochondrial lipids were extracted with a mixture of chloroform: methanol (2:1). The amount of individual phospholipid fractions was determined by the method of flow horizontal chromatography (Kargapolov, 1981). The precipitate on the filter was washed three times with a mixture of chloroform - methanol (2:1) I ml each and hot methanol. Treatment with methanol favours better extraction of lysophospholipids as well as acidic phospholipids (Kargapolov et al., 1975). To the filtrate, 2-3 ml of 0.2% calcium chloride solution was added until two phases were formed: chloroform and water-methanol. The tubes were then shaken for 1-2 min and 2 ml of chloroform was added. After clear separation, the upper phase was sucked off. The lipids remaining in the upper phase were extracted with 2 ml of chloroform. The combined chloroform extract was washed three times with a chloroform-methanol-0.02%CaCI $mixture_2$ (3:48:47). After washing, 1/10 of the available volume was withdrawn for determination of total lipid phosphorus (Baginskietal., 1967). The remaining lipid extract was evaporated to dryness in a nitrogen current and dissolved in 20-25 µl of chloroform-methanol mixture (2:1).

KSK silica gel was used as an adsorbent for thin-layer chromatography. The adsorbent was applied to a 24x9 cm plate by precipitation method (Kargapolov and Kartseva, 1975). The plates were air-dried, then activated in a desiccator at 120°C for 15 minutes and separated into 10-15 separate tracks with a width of 4-5 mm using a special device. The studied lipid material in the amount of 10-40 µg in the volume of 2-5 µl was applied to plates placed in flat glass chambers for flow chromatography. Phospholipids were fractionated in chloroform-methanol-ammonia system (12.4:4.6:1.0). Chromatograms after drying were exposed directly over the chromium mixture in a special vessel placed in a desiccator at 200°C^0 for 30 min. After the chromatograms were shown, the quantitative content of individual lipid fractions was determined by densitometry (Novitskaya, 1972).

2. 6. Disc electrophoresis of mitochondrial membrane proteins.

Disc electrophoresis was performed in 11% polyacrylamide gel according to the method of Neville and Clossmann (1971). The concentrating gel was 3% PAGE. Mitochondria were dissolved in extraction medium containing sodium dodecyl sulfate and -mercaptoethanol to a final concentration of 1%, incubated in this mixture at 37°C for I hour. Sodium dodecyl sulfate (SDS) was purified from impurities of inorganic salts by two-fold recrystallisation from 70% ethanol followed by two-fold washing of dry SDS with hot butyl alcohol. Impurities of hydrocarbons and alcohols were removed by two-fold extraction with ethyl ether. The first 30 min electrophoresis was carried out at a current of 2 mA per tube, then the current was increased to 5 mA per tube. 0.05% bromo-phenol blue was used as a marker dye. After elecrophoresis, gels were fixed for 20 minutes in 10% TCA. Gels were stained in 0.25% Coomassie R-250 prepared on a methanol-acetic acid-water mixture (5:7:78). Densitometry was performed on a Karl Zeiss densitometer (Jena, GDR).

2. 7. Reactants.

The following reagents were used in the work: ADP, ATP, Nad.H succinic acid, histidine, EDTA (Reanal-Hungary), cytochrome c (Biomed-Poland), rotenone (sigma-USA), ascorbic acid, glutamic acid, 2,4-DNF, sucrose, tris, BSA - mark "B", inorganic salts and other reagents of b.h. and b.d.a. qualification (Reachim-Russia). Reanal (Benrpna) reagent kits were used for disc electrophoresis.

2.8. Statistical processing of the results.

All data were processed statistically using the formula:

$$\sigma = \sqrt{\frac{\sum x^2}{(n-1)}}$$

where is the mean square deviation, x n is the number of experiments.

The reliability of the obtained data was calculated using the formula:

$$M_1 - M_2 \geq \sqrt{m_1^2 + m_2^2}$$

where M1 is the arithmetic mean of the experiment, M_2 is the arithmetic mean of the control, m1 is the mean error of the experiment, m_2 is the mean error of the control.

Chapter 3

RESEARCH RESULTS AND THEIR DISCUSSION.

3.1. Comparative study of respiration and oxidative phosphorylation of liver mitochondria of pregnant rabbits, embryos and placenta under the action of butyphos during embryonic development.

At present, there is quite unambiguous literature data indicating the high sensitivity of mitochondria to various chemical and physical effects directed to the tissues of the whole organism. There is a basis for the statement that mitochondria are the most sensitive part of the cell, and their reactions and state determine the reactions and state of the whole cell (Kondrashova, 1968).

Mitochondria possess all basic functions of the cell (Sku-lachev, 1969) and, therefore, the response of isolated mitochondria - their metabolic states - should correspond to the general physiological laws of response of living entities to external influences. As we noted in the Literature Review, it is the mitochondria and mitochondrial energy transformation apparatus that may represent the primary intracellular target for many pesticides.

It is known, however, that during pregnancy physiological changes occur in the organism aimed at the preservation of the embryo and its further development. The totality of changes in the maternal organism can have numerous influences on the realisation of the effects of chemical agents that have entered it from the environment. In this regard, it is of interest to compare the functions of maternal and foetal liver mitochondria during butifos poisoning.

Administration of butifos to rabbits resulted on the 23rd day of gestation in an average 20% decrease in the rate of succinate oxidation by the liver mitochondria of rabbits in the V4 state, while the rate of ADP and DNF-stimulated respiration practically did not differ from the control (Table 1). As a result of such changes, the conjugation of mitochondrial preparations, assessed by the magnitude of DC, increased; a slight increase in the ADP/O ratio was also noted. Similar changes under the influence of butyphos were observed in mitochondria when glutamate was used as a substrate. In this oxidation of glutamate in the V state$_4$ npaKTH4ecKn does not change, but the rate of phosphorylation respiration of mitochondria slightly increased, which also led to a slight increase in the value of respiratory control. In parallel, the rate of DNF-stimulated respiration of mitochondria also increased. The above means, apparently, that the introduction of butyphos into animals at 23 pregnancies induces changes in mitochondria that contribute to a decrease in "basal" passive membrane permeability, as evidenced by a decrease in respiration in the V state$_4$.

The rate of succinate oxidation in mitochondria isolated from the liver of experimental rabbits (30 days of embryonic development) in the metabolic states V_4 n $Vj|_{I(I)}$ does not differ from the control, single inhibited by 14% in the state V_3 (Table 1). Although the liver mitochondria of experimental rabbits are characterised by inhibition of respiration in the metabolic state V_3 , the rate of succinate oxidation upon addition of the uncoupler remains high, indicating that there is no direct effect of butifos on the respiratory chain. These mitochondrial preparations of glutamate oxidation under different metabolic states are characterised by slightly reduced respiratory activity. At the same time, the value of DA tends to decrease and the ADP/O ratio increases.

Table 1.

Effect of treatment of pregnant rabbits with butifos on respiration and oxidative phosphorylation of maternal liver mitochondria (MH$_{мат}$), placental mitochondria (MH$_{ПЛ}$) and embryonic liver mitochondria (MH$_{эмб}$.) at 23 and 30 days of development.

(Respiration rate is in ng atom O_2 /min.mg protein. Oxidation substrate - succinate, V_4 * - respiration rate before addition of ADP. Table represents Mim, number of experiments 5-7; k - control, o - experiment).

Indicator	mh$_{мат}$		MX™		mh$_{эмб}$.	
	к	о	к	о	к	о
23 days						
V4*	23±2	18±1	7±0,1	9,6±0,2	23±3	24±4
V3	67±4	64±2	16,5±0,6	18,0±0,5	47±3	62±4
V4	26±2	21±1	7,5±0,2	10,0±0,3	20±2	22±2
UDNF	72±2	74±2	14,0±0,4	16,7±0,3	52±3	67±2
dk	2,6±0,1	3,0±0,06	2,3±0,05	1,9±0,03	2,4±0,01	2,8±0,1
ADP/O	1,8±0,03	1,9±0,04	1,8±0,06	1,6±0,09	1,7±0,06	1,9±0,05
30 days						
V4*	23±1	23±2	7,5±0,2	4,6 ±0,4	30±2	25±1
V3	80±3	69±2	16,0±0,1	12,7±0,4	74±5	63±2
V4	29±1	28±2	7,8±0,2	4,4±0,1	30±3	29±2
UDNF	85±4	81±4	16,8±0,4	13,0±0,2	85±4	60±3
DK	2,8±0,03	2,4±0,03	2,0±0,03	2,9±0,06	2,5±0,06	2,2±0,01
ADP/O	1,7±0,02	2,0±0,1	1,8±0,1	1,9±0,06	1,8±0,06	1,6±0,03

Mitochondria isolated from the placenta of experimental rabbits are characterised by an increased rate of succinate oxidation in various metabolic states, especially - V_4 (by 33%). At the same time, the value of ADP/O was reduced by 11.2% and DC by 17% compared to the control (Table 1). Since the decrease of ADP/O ratio and DC value (according to Chance) was accompanied in our experiments by the increase of respiration rate in V_4 oho state was obviously connected with dissociation of oxidative phosphorylation.

Mitochondria from the placenta on the 30th day of pregnancy were characterised in the experiment by a reduced rate of succinate oxidation in various metabolic states. The decrease in respiration was particularly marked in state V_4 (by 44%), leading to an increase in the value of respiratory control. The value of ADP/O coefficient also tended to increase.

Administration of butyphos to rabbits induced changes in respiration and oxidative phosphorylation in fetal liver mitochondria as well. On day 23 of embryo development, an increase in the rate of succinate oxidation was observed in various metabolic states. The acceleration of mitochondrial respiration in the metabolic state V_3 (na 32%) was particularly marked, accompanied by a 16.6% increase in DA value. A similar increase was also observed in media with glutamate. The ADP/O ratio in media with succinate increased by 11.7% compared to the control and by 16% for glutamate oxidation (Table 1).

In the model we used, we studied relatively remote (10-day period) biochemical consequences of treatment of animals with mild doses (1/20 LD_{50}) of butifos. It is clear that under these conditions direct effects of the studied pesticide on mitochondria functions can be excluded, and the measured parameters of their functional state obviously reflect changes in the number of respiratory transporters and (or) activity of the systems of transport of respiration and phosphorylation substrates through the inner membrane of mitochondria. Modification of the lipid microenvironment of membrane-bound enzymes may play an important functional role under these conditions. In general, the changes in the parameters of oxidative phosphorylation of placenta, maternal liver and embryo induced by low doses of butyphos described in this section are apparently compensatory and tissue-specific in nature. Changes in the activity of the oxidative phosphorylation process are most intense on the 30th day in the mitochondria of the embryo and placenta liver compared to the mitochondria of the mother's liver. This indicates the embryotropic effect of low doses of butifos, which undoubtedly has a complex nature including modification of mitochondrial functions.

3. 2. Effect of butifos on the activity of oxidase systems of mitochondrial membranes of liver mitochondria, embryo placenta and maternal liver.

In recent years, considerable experimental material has been accumulated on changes in the activity of membrane-bound enzymes and polyenzyme systems of mitochondria under the action of various factors and drugs. The study of the effect of pesticides on the functioning of the mitochondrial respiratory chain is one of the most important tests used in deciphering the primary mechanisms of intoxication. The task of the present section was to comparatively study the effect of butifos on the activity of oxidase systems of mitochondria membranes of liver, placenta of embryos and maternal liver.

If in experiments on intact mitochondria the observed inhibition of respiration can be a consequence of both disturbances directly in the respiratory chain and in the system of substrate transport through the inner membrane, then in the case of preparations of frozen-thawed mitochondria the latter factor is not rate-limiting.

Preparations of mitochondria subjected to single freezing and thawing were used in these experiments. The level of mitochondrial succinatoxidase activity from the above-mentioned organs and tissues of animals under the action of butifos at a dose of 1/20 LD_{50} is presented in Figures 3 and 4. The value of succinatoxidase activity under butifos exposure decreased in mitochondria of placenta and liver of pregnant rabbits, especially on the 30th day of embryo development (Figs. 36, 46). At the same time, butifos markedly activated the succinatoxidase system of the respiratory chain of embryos. Its activity on the 23rd day of embryo development was increased by 24.5%, and on the 30th day - by 19.5% compared to the control (Fig. 3a, 4a).

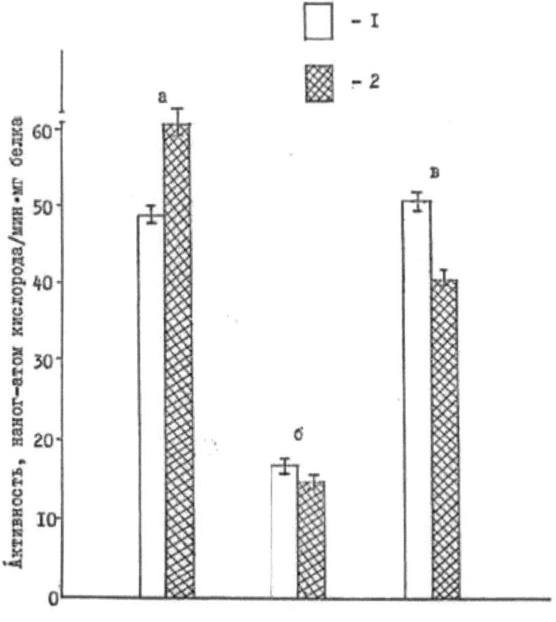

Figure 3. SUCCINATOXIDASE ACTIVITY LEVELS OF MYTOCHONDRY MITOCHONDRY MITOCHONDRY LIVES OF 23-DAY-OLD EMBRIONS (a), PLACENTA (b) AND BUTIFOS IN CONTROL (1) AND IN THE IMPLICATION OF BUTIFOS (2)

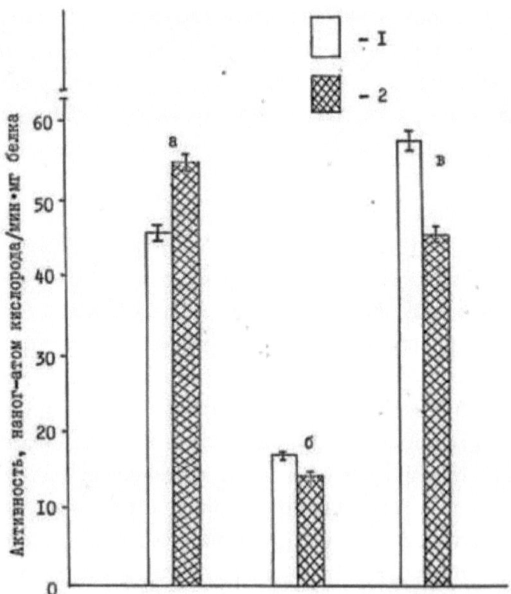

Fig. 4 LEVELS OF SUCCINATOXIDASE ACTIVITY OF MYTOCHONDRY MITOCHONDRY MITOCHONDRIES IN 30-DAY EMBRION, PLACENTA, AND BIRTHY BREAST LIV IN CONTROL (1) AND SUBSTANCE THE EFFECTS OF BUTIFOS
(Designations as in Fig. 3)

Data on NAD.H-xidase activity of mitochondria of embryonic liver, placenta and maternal liver mitochondria during exposure to butifos are presented in Tables 6-8.

It follows from the presented data that butifos poisoning affects the activity of NAD.H-oxidase in different ways: the oxidase activity of mitochondria of embryo liver on the 23rd and 30th days of development increases compared to the control by 17 and 15.8%, respectively (Table 6). At the same time, this oxidase system in mitochondria of placenta and maternal liver decreases its activity as a result of butifos action (Tables 7, 8).

On the 23rd day of embryo development the activity of NAD.H-oxidase system of maternal liver mitochondria decreases by 22%, but on the 30th day of embryo development its activity is gradually restored, but does not reach the control level. It should be noted that under the influence of butifos the greatest decrease in the activity of NAD.H- oxidase is observed in the case of placenta mitochondria, where on the

23rd and 30th day of embryo development the activity decreases by 36.4 and 28.6%, respectively, against the control level (Table 7).

It is known that liver mitochondria have two oxidation systems (Fig. 2) - an internal phosphorylation pathway for oxidation of NAD-dependent substrates, and an external pathway for free oxidation of added NAD.H (Fig. 2). The initial part of the respiratory chain of this pathway is NAD-N-cytochrome-in_5 -reductase (Skulachev, 1969;Raw, Makier, 1959).Destruction of mitochondria by freezing and thawing leads to loss of conjugation, but retains the ability to oxidise NAD.H through the mitochondrial external (rotenone-insensitive) and internal (rotenone-sensitive) pathways.

Table 6.

Effect of butyphos on NAD.H-oxidase activity and its nature after the addition of cytochrome c in mitochondria.

isolated from the liver of embryos (M±m)

(k - control. o - experience)

Gestational age, days	Variant	Activity, nanog-atom of oxygen / mn^mig of protein								
		NADPH oxidase			Rothenon-insensitive NADPH oxidase			Ротенон-чувствительная NADPH oxidase		
		NAD.H	NADZN + Cite.c	YES	NAD.H	NADZN + Cite.c	YES	NADC	NAD.H + Cite.c	YES
23	к	35±2	134±6	99	18±1	110±3	92	17±1	24±3	7
	0	41±2	163+8	122	22±1	143±5	121	19±1	20±3	-
		£<0,001	£<0,001		£<0,001	£<0,001		£<0,1	£<0,002	
30	к	38±2	149+8	111	20±1	115±5	95	18±1	34±3	16
	0	44±2	167±9	123	24±1	138±6	114	20±1	29±3	9
		£<0,001	£<0,001		£<0,001	£<0,001		£<0-01	£<0,001	

Effect of buty f os on NADLH oxidase activity and its p r o d u c t i o n after addition of cytochrome c in mitochondria.

isolated from the liver of embryos

(k - control o - experience)

Gestational age, days	Variant	Activity, nanog-atom of oxygen/min.mg protein								
		N AD. N o k s i d a za			Rotenon gjUuU eUlitelny n ADLf-o k sida za			Rotenon DUvideteln na me N ADL- oK CИ E a за		
		NADLCH	NADL + Cited from.	YES	NADH	NADL + Cited from.	YES	NADL	NADL + Cited from.	YES
23	К	22+1	57+3	35	8+0,5	43±2	35	14±0,5	14,5±0,5	-
	0	14+1	45+2	31	6 ±0,4	37±2	31	8+0,6	8; 6±0.6	-
		P<0,001	P<0,001		P>0,05	P<0,001		P<0,001	P<0,001	
30	к	21±1	52±3	31	11±1	42±2	31	10±1	10±1	-
	о	15±1	43+3	28	7,5±1	35±2	27,3	7,5±O,5	7,5±0,5	-
		P<0,001	P<0,001		P<0,001	P<0,001		P<0,001	P<0,001	

Table 8.

Effect of butyphos on NAD.H-oxidase activity and its increases after addition of cytochrome a in mitochondria

isolated from embryo liver (M±m)

(k - control, o - experience]

Gestational age, days	Variant	Activity, nanog-atom of oxygen / min.mg protein								
		NADN-o k sida za			Rothenon-insensitive N ADN-o to sid a for			Rotenon-chu NADH oxidase		
		NADH	NAD.H + Cite.c	LA	NADH	NADH + Cit.c	YES	NADH	NAD.H + Cite.c	YES
23	К	36±2	120±8	84	12±1	69+3	57	24±2	51±5	27
	О	28±2	95±5	67	10±1	63+3	53	18+1	32±2	14
		P<0,001	P<0,001		P<0,1	£<0,001		P<0,00!	P<0,001	
30	К	33±2	144+10	111	12+2	74+5	62	21±2	70+4	49
	О	29±2	97±7	68	10±2	63+4	53	19+1	34±3	15
		P<0,001	£<0,001		£<0,05	£<0,001		P<0,05	P<0; 00!	

Administration of butyphos to animals leads to activation (in the case of embryo liver mitochondria) or inhibition (in the case of placenta and rabbit liver mitochondria) of the internal and external pathways of NAD-H oxidation depending on the time of embryo development (Tables 6-8). When analysing the ratio of NAD.H oxidation rates by internal and external oxidation pathways, it can be seen that bu-tifos significantly increases the activity of rotenone-insensitive NAD.H oxidase system of embryo liver mitochondria (Table b). Thus, while the activity of rotenone-insensitive NAD.H-oxidase increases by 20-22%, the activity of NAD.H-oxidase of the rotenone-sensitive pathway increases only by 11-12% compared to the control. At the same time in mitochondria of placenta (Table 7) and maternal liver (Table 8) under the influence of butifos a different picture is observed - suppression of activity of both oxidases, and in mitochondria of rabbits' liver the activity of rotenone-sensitive NAD.H-oxidase is especially markedly suppressed.

Quite interesting data were obtained when studying the effect of butifos on mitochondria of placenta of embryos. Thus, on the 23rd day of embryonic development the activity of rotenone-insensitive NAD.H-oxidase in placenta mitochondria decreases by 25%, at the same time the activity of NAD.H-oxidase of the rotenone-sensitive pathway is suppressed by 43%. However, on the 30th day of embryonic development, the decrease in the activity of these NAD.H oxidation pathways does not reach the level characteristic of mitochondria isolated from the liver of 23-day-old embryos. Thus, analysing the ratio of activities of external and internal pathways of NAD.H oxidation, we can conclude that under the influence of butifos, the activity of rotenone-insensitive NAD.H-oxidase of mitochondria of embryo liver is mainly increased and, on the contrary, the activity of rotenone-sensitive NAD.H-oxidase of the respiratory chain of mitochondria of placenta and maternal liver is markedly suppressed (Tables 7, 8).

It is known that membrane disorders associated with pathologies and changes in phospholipid and protein composition significantly alter the ability of exogenous cytochrome c to activate electron transfer along the respiratory chain (Rakhimov and Almatov, 1978; Almatov et al, 1981,1982).This is manifested, on the one hand, in changes in the activity of cytochrome c-oxidase, for which cytochrome c is a substrate, and, on the other hand, in the magnitude of increases in NAD.H-oxidase and succinatoxidase activities observed when exogenous cytochrome c is introduced into the reaction medium. These characteristics are very sensitive to the presence of "hidden damage" of mitochondrial membranes as a result of pathological process or during the action of damaging factors. Thus, they can serve as a reliable test indicating the state of polyenzyme systems of mitochondrial membranes. In this connection, we studied the interaction of exogenous cytochrome c with mitochondria of the liver of embryonic foetuses, placenta and liver of pregnant rabbits. As can be seen from Figures 5 and 6, a deviation of cytochrome c-oxidase activity from the control level is observed under the action of butifos. The most noticeable changes are observed on the 30th day of embryo development. Thus, the activity of cytochrome-c-oxidase of mitochondria of rabbit liver on the 23rd day of embryo development does not change significantly, but on the 30th day it decreases by 23%. A similar decrease in cytochrome-c-oxidase activity under the influence of butifos occurs in mitochondria isolated from the placenta of embryos, while the activity of cytochrome-c-oxidase of mitochondria

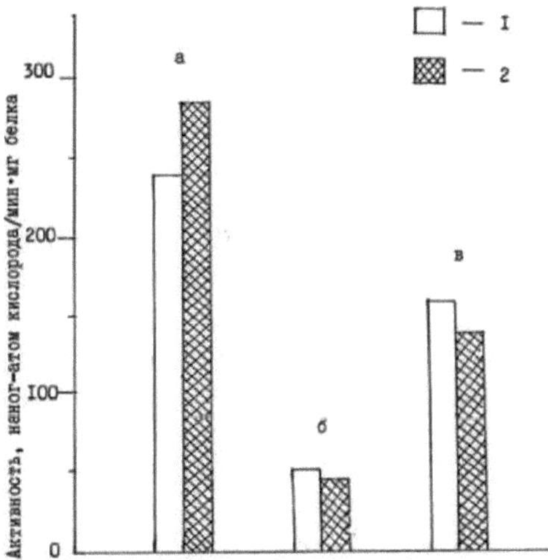

Figure 5. ACTIVITY OF CYTOCHROME C-OXIDASE OF MITOCHONDRIA OF LIVER MITOCHONDRIA OF 23-DAY EMBRYOS, PLACENTA AND LIVER OF PREGNANT RABBITS IN CONTROL (I) AND UNDER THE INFLUENCE OF BUTIFOS (2).

(Designation as in Fig. 3)

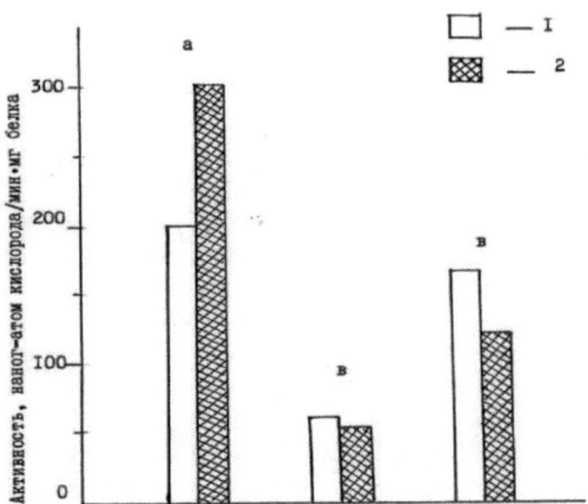

Figure 6. ACTIVITY LEVEL OF CYTOCHROME C-OXIDASE OF MITOCHONDRIA
LIVER OF 30-DAY EMBRYOS, PLACENTA AND LIVER OF PREGNANT RABBITS IN CONTROL (I) AND UNDER THE INFLUENCE OF BUTIFOSA(2). (Designation as in Fig. 3)

liver of embryos increases, especially noticeable on the 30th day of embryo development. Thus, if the activity of this enzymatic system on the 23rd day of embryo development increases by 16.6%, on the 30th day - by 39% of the control level.

Thus, our studies suggest that butifos has different effects on the oxidase systems of mitochondrial membranes of liver, embryos, placenta and maternal liver. Thus, if butifos leads to an increase in the rate of electron transfer along the respiratory chain in the mitochondria of the embryo liver, then in the mitochondria of the placenta and maternal liver, on the contrary, this process slows down under the influence of butifos. It can be considered that two types of disturbances in the structure of mitochondria of the studied organs take place during butifos poisoning. One of them is manifested in the change of structural "conjugation" between separate parts of the respiratory chain, and the second one is caused by degradation of the whole respiratory chain and the external pathway of NAD.H oxidation.

As it was noted, under the influence of butifos the activity of poly- enzyme systems of mitochondria of the liver of embryos increases, while in mitochondria of placenta and maternal liver it decreases. These observations are in agreement with the data obtained by other authors during the study of various pathological processes in their mild stages, in which an increase in the rate of substrate oxidation was usually observed, possibly due to an improvement in the diffusion of substrates to the active centres of the corresponding poly-enzyme systems, as a result of the formation of "hidden damage" in the structure of mitochondrial membranes. At deeper degrees of pathology, the marked processes were transformed into inactivation processes, which is associated with deeper damage to the inner membrane of mitochondria (Almatov et al., 1981, 1982; Agzamov et al., 1981, 1983; Rakhimov, Almatov, 1977; Musaev et al., 1981).

3.8. The effect of butifos on the activation of the NAD.H-oxidase system of mitochondrial membranes by cytochrome c.

The addition of cytochrome c to the medium containing dissociated mitochondria and NAD.H increases the rate of electron transfer along the respiratory chain. It is known that cytochrome c can be incorporated into membrane phospholipids, forming electrostatic bonds with them (Ivanetichetal., 1974). The incorporation of exogenous cytochrome c is very sensitive to the structural coupling between proteins and phospholipids of the mitochondrial inner membrane (Almatov, et al., 1982). Changes in mitochondrial membranes caused by exposure of the organism to stress factors or pathological processes lead to disruption of "inclusion "* of exogenous cytochrome c in the mitochondrial membrane, i.e. activation of the polyenzyme systems of the mitochondrial respiratory chain by cytochrome c is impaired.

It follows from the results shown in Tables 6-8 that the total rate of NAD.H oxidation after the addition of cytochrome c to the polarographic cell is different in mitochondria of control and experimental animals. Meanwhile, the total NAD.H-oxidase activity of mitochondria of placenta and maternal liver of experimental animals does not reach the level of control (Tables 7, 8). At the same time, in mitochondria of the liver of embryos injected with butifos, the activity of this system is markedly increased (Table b). However, if we calculate how many times the rate of NAD-H oxidation changes after the addition of cytochrome c, we observe a different car-

*The term "inclusion" is very conventional and means in experiments of this type the activating effect of exogenous cytochrome c on oxidase systems. It is clear that the direct incorporation of cytochrome c into mitochondrial membranes is not always a rate-limiting process in the electron transfer chain.

tin. At the same time, a greater degree of increase in the activity of NAD.H-oxidase of placenta mitochondria is observed in the experiment compared to the control. In particular, on the 23rd day of embryo development the activity after addition of cytochrome c in the control increases 2.59 times, but in animals receiving butifos - 3.21 times. At the same time, the degree of increase of NAD.H-oxidase activity after addition of cytochrome c in mitochondria of liver of embryos and maternal organism in the experiment does not differ from the control. On the 30th day of embryo development in the mitochondria of the liver of the maternal organism (Table 8), the increase in activity after the addition of cytochrome c in the experiment (butifos) is lower than in the control.

A comparative study of NAD.H oxidation in media containing cytochrome c + rotenone showed that cytochrome c mainly accelerates electron transfer along the external pathway of mitochondrial oxidation; this agrees with the data of other studies (Skulachev, 1969; Rakhimov and Almatov, 1978; Almatov et al., 1982). The presence of exogenous cytochrome in the medium is an indispensable condition for the activation of the external oxidation pathway. It follows from the data presented in Tables 6-8 that butifos inoculation on day 23 of embryo development causes an increase in the activity of rotenone-insensitive NAD.H-oxidase (in the presence of cytochrome c) of the mitochondria of the embryo liver, but simultaneously in the mitochondria of all tissues, especially in the case of the mother's liver, the activity of the rotenone-sensitive NAD.H-oxidase system of mitochondria in media with cytochrome c is markedly suppressed. It should be noted that exogenous cytochrome c practically does not activate the rotenone-sensitive NAD.H-oxidase system of mitochondria of placenta of embryos both in the control and in the experiment (Table 7).

On the 30th day of embryo development under the influence of butifos the activity of rotenone-insensitive NAD .H-oxidase (in the presence of cytochrome c) system of embryo liver mitochondria slightly increases (Table 6) and tends to decrease in mitochondria of placenta and maternal liver (Tables 7, 8).

The study of the effect of butifos inoculation on the activity of the ro-tenon-sensitive NAD.H-oxidase system shows that on the 30th day of embryo development, as well as in the case of earlier developmental periods, suppression of the activity of this system is observed in media with exogenous cytochrome c, especially clearly in the case of maternal liver mitochondria (Table 8).

From the above, we can make a general conclusion that during the action of butifos on the organism of pregnant animals, "hidden damages" are formed in the structure of mitochondria of liver mitochondria of embryos, placenta and liver of the maternal organism. The authors of this term (Almatov et al., 1981,1982) suggest that they are based on the disturbance of interactions between proteins and lipids in the mitochondrial membrane. On the other hand, it is possible that under the influence of pathology, poisoning or stress, the amount, availability and/or activity of lytic enzymes is altered both in mitochondria themselves and in lysosomes present in the mitochondrial fraction. These "lesions" are manifested by impaired rates of oxidation and phosphorylation, activity of polyenzyme systems, and access of exogenous cytochrome squ to the appropriate regions of mitochondrial membranes. The presented data indicate that under the influence of butifos on the organism of pregnant animals there are observed rather deep disturbances in the system of oxidative phosphorylation and electron transfer chain in mitochondria of the liver of embryos, placenta and liver of the maternal organism, especially at later terms of pregnancy.

3.9. Phospholipid composition of mitochondrial membranes of liver mitochondria of embryos, placenta and liver of pregnant rabbits in normal and under the influence of butifos.

It is well known that the action of organophosphorus pesticides on biological membranes is based on inhibition of cholinesterases. Recently, however, information is beginning to accumulate that in the pathogenesis of intoxication with compounds of this class their interaction with biological membranes, i.e. their membranotoxic effect, plays a certain role; the manifestation of this effect may include an increase in membrane permeability, the development of hyperfermentemia (Dolgo-Saburov, 1969) and disruption of membrane-bound enzymes (Ivanova et al., 1978; Mirakhmedov et al., 1984; Khamidov et al., 1984).Mirahmedov et al.,1984; Khamidov et al.,1984; Sheraliev et al.,1984; Kleshgok, Rajtor, 1979).

An essential integral component of biological membranes is phospholipids, which ensure their normal functional activity and control of lipid-dependent enzymes. On the basis of few data it can be concluded that intoxication with organophosphorus pesticides is accompanied by quantitative and qualitative changes in the lipid composition of membranes (Gerickeetal., 1976; Hettwer,Gericke, 1977). As is known, quantitative changes in phospholipids are accompanied by disorders of microstructure, physicochemical properties and basic functions of membranes, in particular, the strength, conductivity, enzymatic activity, selective permeability of these structures with respect to various metabolites, cations and anions are significantly altered.

There are no studies devoted to studying the effect of pesticides, in particular, organophosphorus compounds, on the quantitative and qualitative content of individual phospholipid fractions in mitochondria of embryonic tissues. The study of cell phospholipid content, in particular, mitochondria of animal organs in the mother-placenta-fetus system contributes to the elucidation of the mechanism of pesticide-induced energy function disorders in cells. In this connection, it was of interest to investigate the changes of major and minor fractions of phospholipids in mitochondria of maternal, foetal and rabbit liver and placenta under the action of butifos.

The results of studies on the effect of butifos on the phospholipid composition of liver mitochondria of pregnant rabbits are shown in Tables 9 and 10.

As can be seen from the data obtained, the phospholipid composition of liver mitochondria of pregnant rabbits changes in response to the action of butifos. In the process of studying the effect of butifos on the phospholipid composition of mitochondria of this organ very significant changes were found. In particular, on the 23rd and 30th days of pregnancy there was an increase in the content of phosphatidylcholine (by 9.6 and 9.7 per cent), phosphatidylethanolamine (by 11.4 and 17.6 per cent), phosphatidylinositol (by 7.7 and 37.5 per cent), phosphatidylserine (by 25.0 and 37.5 per cent), phosphatidic acid (by 13.3 and 28,5%) and lysophosphatidic acid (by 12.5 and 11.7%) with simultaneous decrease of cardiolipin (by 32.0 and 38.7%), sphingomyelin (by 12.3 and 27.7%), lysophosphatidylcholine (by 9.6 and 20.0%), lysophosphatidylethanolamine (by 12.3 and 17.0%) and lysocardiolipin (by 20.0 and 50.0%) relative to control. Apparently, under the action of butifos in different liver compartments methylation reactions are accelerated (conversion of phosphatidyl ethanolamine to phosphatidylcholine), decarboxylation (conversion of phosphatidylserine to phosphatidylethanolamine) and base exchange (ethanolamine, serine, inositol) (Bereziat, 1980). On the other hand,

Table 9

Percentage content of separate fractions of phospholipids in mitochondria of rabbit liver on 23 days of pregnancy in normal and under the action of butifos (M + t, n= 5-7).

Phospholipids	Control	Experience
Phosphatidylcholine	33,2±1,4	36,4±2,3
Phosphatidylethanolamine	25,4+1,3	28,3±2,0
Cardiolipin	15,6±1,6	10,6±1,0
Phosphatidylserine	2,8±2	3,5±0,1
Phosphatidylinositol	I,3±0,1	1,4±0,I
Sphingomyelin	4,9±0,5	4,3±0,2
Phosphatidic acid	I,5±0,1	1,7±0,2
Lysophosphatidylcholine	2,1±0,1	1,9=0,04
Lysophosphatidylethanolamine	10,6±0,6	9,3=0,9
Lysocardiolipin	1,0=0,02	0,8=0,01
Lysophosphatidic acid	1,6±),1	I,8=0,3

increase in the content of acidic phospholipids - phosphatidylserine, phosphatidylinositol in response to butyphos action is a defence reaction of the organism. Acidic phospholipids are known to be functionally very important, although they are contained in relatively small amounts in mitochondrial membranes (Bruni, Toffano, 1982; Painetal..., 1983; Agranoff, 1983).The marked increase in phosphatidylserine and phosphatidylinositol content in rabbit liver mitochondria after the action of butyphos appears to be important because these phospholipid fractions, especially phosphatidylserine, are able to exert a significant effect on membrane-bound enzymes (Shvets et al., 1974; Rybalchenko et al., 1974),

Table 10

Percentage content of separate fractions of phospholipids in mitochondria of rabbit liver on 30 days of pregnancy in norm and under the action of butifos (M + m, n = 5-7).

Phospholipids	Control	Experience
Phosphatidylcholine	34,0±1,5	37,3±1,4
Phosphatidylethanolamine	25,0±1,2	29,4±2,4
Cardiolipin	15,6±1,3	9,5+0,8
Phosphatidylserine	3,2±),2	4,4±),8
Phosphatidylinositol	I,2±0,1	I,8±0,1
Sphingomyelin	4,7±0,5	3,4±),2
Phosphatidic acid	I,4±0,1	1,8±0,2
Lysophosphatidylcholine	2,1+0,1	1,6=0,05
Lysophosphatidylethanolamine	10,0±0,8	8,3±),6
Lysocardiolipin	1,2±),02	0,6±0,02
Lysophosphatidic acid	I,7±0,1	I,9±0,1

1977; Bruni, Toffano, 1982).

It is known that cardiolipin is of great importance in the organisation of mitochondrial membranes, and while phosphatidi- lcholine and phosphatidylethanolamine are relatively easily removed from mitochondrial membranes, cardiolipin, on the contrary, is firmly bound to them and is not removed under the influence of even strong organic solvents (Awasthietal., 1971; Berezneyetal., 1970). In mitochondria, these lipids play a significant role as factors involved in the regulation of the activity of respiratory chain enzymes and ion transport. In particular, it has been shown that cleavage of cardiolipins is accompanied by inhibition of cytochrome oxidase activity (Zahier and Fieisher, 1971). Reduction of cardiolipins as a result of butifos action is accompanied by a sharp increase in the minor component of mitochondrial lipids - phosphatidylserines and phosphatidylinositols, which indicates increased synthesis of these compounds, possibly as a result of the reaction of interconversions of individual phospholipids characteristic of mitochondria (Vgesheg, Greenberg, 1961; Gibsonetal.,1961). It can be concluded that butyphos in maternal liver mitochondria inhibits cardiolipin biosynthesis.

It is known that lyso-derivatives of phospholipids are products of partial degradation of phospholipids. By measuring the amounts of lyso-derivatives, it is possible to judge to some extent the degradation rates of phospholipids. As is known, phospholipid lyso derivatives play an important role in the function of biological membranes and are formed in these cell organelles as a result of activation of endogenous phospholipases under certain functional conditions. (Kargapolov, 1979; Parceetal, 1978; Gan-Elepano, Meal, 1978; chan, Higgins, 1978). In this connection, in order to identify the causes of changes in the content of phospholipids, we studied the content of lysoforms of certain phospholipids of rabbit liver mitochondria under the action of butifos. The obtained results indicate that under the influence of this pesticide all lysophospholipids, except for lysophosphatidic acid, are broken down .

lysophospholipids, apparently, is a protective mechanism, since it is known that their excessive amount contributes to the disruption of the structure of biological membranes (Hunteretal., 1974). However, it has also been shown that lysophospholipids, and especially lysocardiolipin, which is a carrier of potassium ions (Evtodienko et al., 1977), play an important role in the transport of ions across the mitochondrial membrane. Therefore, the presence in mitochondria of endogenous phospholipases and

lysophospholipases, apparently, provide regulation of oxidative phosphorylation and permeability of mitochondrial membranes, maintaining the necessary level of lysocardiolipins ,

lysophosphatidylethanolamines and lysophosphatidylcholines and their diacyl forms in the mitochondrial membrane.

Under the action of butifos, a parallel increase in the content of phosphatidic acid, as well as its lyso-form, apparently indicates stimulation of both biosynthesis and decomposition of phosphatidic acid. The phosphatidylcholine/phosphatidyleth-anolamine ratio, which plays an important role in membrane structures, is not significantly altered. However, changes were found in the ratio of diacyl forms of phospholipids and their lyso-derivatives. As a result of butifos action in maternal liver mitochondria the phosphatidylcholine/lysophosphatidylcholine ratio increases by 1.22 and 1.37 times, and the phosphatidyl ethanolamine/lysophosphatidylethanolamine ratio by 1.27 and 1.42 times, respectively, on days 23 and 30 of embryonic development. At the same time, the cardiolipin/lysocardiolipin ratio decreases by 15% on the 23rd day of embryonic development, and in contrast, increases by 23% on the 30th day. Consequently, the effect of butyphos is characterised by changes in the ratio of lyso- and diacyl forms specific for each form of phospholipids.

Analysing the results of studies on the effect of butifos on phospholipids of embryo liver mitochondria membranes, it should be noted that on the 23rd and 30th days of embryonic development there is an increase in the content of phosphatidylcholine by 9 and 15%, phosphatidylethanolamine by 8 and 14%, phosphatidylserine by 80 and 63%, and phosphatidic acid by 15 and 31%, respectively, relative to the control (Tables II and 12). In contrast to the above-mentioned

Table II.

Percentage content of individual phospholipid fractions in liver mitochondria of 23-day embryos in normal and at

Butyphos action (M dm, n = 5-7).

Phospholipids	Control	Experience
Phosphatidylcholine	38,1+1,3	41,5+1,8
Phosphatidylethanolamine	27,4+1,2	29,6+2,3
Cardiolipin	10,5+0,5	8,9+0,7
Phosphatidylserine	2,5+0,2	4,5+0,4
Phosphatidylinositol	1,5+0,1	1,2+0,07
Sphingomyelin	4,0+0,3	3,0+0,3
Phosphatidic acid	1,3+0,05	1,7+0,07
Lysophosphatidylcholine	3,0+0,4	2,7+0,1
Lysophosphatidylethanolamine	8,4+0,7	6,4+0,5
Lysocardiolipin	2,1+0,1	1,1+0,08
Lysophosphatidic acid	I,4+0,1	0,6+0,01

The level of cardiolipins, phosphatidylinositols and sphingomyelins decreased on the 23rd day of development by 15 and 25%, and on the 30th day - by 30 and 51%, respectively, from the control level. The observed changes in the content of phospholipids should be considered as a result of disturbances in the processes of their metabolism. One of the possible reasons for accumulation of some phospholipids may be an increase in the synthesis of these phospholipids or inhibition of the activity of endogenous phospholipases as a result of butifos action. The most pronounced increase in phosphatidylserine content under butyphos action indicates stimulation of its biosynthesis or its inhibition

Table 12.

Percentage content of individual phospholipid fractions in liver mitochondria of 30-day embryos in normal and at Butyphos action (M $\pm_{T1}$, n= 5-7).

Phospholipids	Control	Experience
Phosphatidylcholine	37,2±1,5	42,8±2,6
Phosphatidylethanolamine	26,3±1,3	30,0±2,1
Cardiolipin	11,2±),8	7,8±0,9
Phosphatidylserine	3,0±0,2	4,9±),6
Phosphatidylinositol	I,7±0,1	1,1±0,09
Sphingomyelin	4,1±0,4	2,0±0,1
Phosphatidic acid	1,3±),07	I,7±0,3
Lysophosphatidylcholine	3,3±),4	2,4±0,2
Lysophosphatidylethanolamine	8,3±),5	5,5±0,07
Lysocardiolipin	2,0±0,1	I,3±0,1
Lysophosphatidic acid	1,6±3,01	0,50,01

its degradation. At the same time, the decrease in the content of other phospholipid fractions, such as cardiolipin, phosphatidylinositol and sphingomyelin, seems to be associated with a decrease in their synthesis or activation of specific phospholipases. The decrease in cardiolipin content in maternal and fetal liver mitochondria may be due to a decrease in unsaturated fatty acids. Such an assumption is supported by the data of Rososetal. (1980), who found a decrease in the level of unsaturated fatty acids when exposed to pesticides.

The study of the content of phospholipid lysophospholipids shows that under the experimental conditions in embryo liver mitochondria there is a decrease in the content of all lysophospholipids studied by us. This indicates activation of lysophospho-lipase activity under the influence of butyphos or weakening of phospholipase activity of liver mitochondrial membranes. The most significant decrease is observed in the case of the fraction of lysocardiolipins, lysophosphatidic acid and lysophosphatidylethanolamines, the content of which decreases against the control level by 47.6 and 35.0%, 57.2 and 68.8%, 23.8 and 33.8%, respectively, at 23 and 30 days of embryonic development. At the same time, the phosphotidylcholine/phosphatidylethanolamine ratio in the liver mitochondria of embryos and experimental animals does not differ from the control. At the same time, changes in the ratio of diacyl forms of phospholipids and their lyso derivatives were detected. As a result of butyphos action the phosphatidylcholine/lysophosphatidylcholine ratio increases in relation to control in 1.2 and 1.6 times, phospha- tidylethanolamine/lysophosphatidylethanolamine in 1.4 and 1.7 times, and phosphatidic acid/lysophosphatidic acid in 2.7 and 4.2 times, respectively on 23 and 30 days of embryo development. The cardiolipin/lysocardiolipin ratio increases 1.6-fold only on day 23 of embryo development, and on day 30 this index does not differ from the control. Consequently, the effect of butyphos on the lipid composition of embryo liver mitochondrial membranes, as in the case of maternal liver mitochondria, is characterised by changes in the ratio of lyso- and diacyl forms specific for each form of phospholipids.

The study of the phospholipid composition of placental mitochondria is highly relevant both with respect to understanding the mechanism of permeability to the pesticide and the effect of butifos on the foetus.

The results of the study showed that butifos had a selective effect on the content of certain fractions of phospholipids of mitochondria of embryonic placenta mitochondria (Tables 13 and 14).

Table 13.

Percentage content of individual phospholipid fractions in mitochondria of rabbit placenta on the 23rd day of pregnancy in normal and under the action of butifos (M djm, n= 5-7).

Phospholipids	Control	Experience
Phosphatidylcholine	41,4±3,2	37,4±2,7
Phosphatidylethanolamine	14,2±1,0	10,1±0,9
Cardiolipin	4,6±0,4	12,1±1,2
Phosphatidylserine	6,1±0,2	3,6±),3
Phosphatidylinositol	5,5±0,6	7,4±0,7
Sphingomyelin	8,7±0,4	11,3±0,9
Phosphatidic acid	2,0±0,3	I,3±0,1
Lysophosphotidylcholine	4,2±0,3	1,0±0,01
Lysophosphotidylethanolamine	9,8±1,0	13,4±0,8
Lysocardiolipin	I,2±0,1	
Lysophosphatidic acid	2,3±0,1	I,7±0,1

At the same time there is a decrease in the content of phosphatidylethanolamine (29 and 28%), phosphatidylserine (41 and 53%), phosphatidic acid (35 and 33%) respectively on 23 and 30 days of embryo development. The decrease in the amount of phosphatidylcholine is only 10-11%. Butyphos action markedly increases cardiolipin (163 and 164%), phosphatidylinositol (34.5 and 33.3%) and sphingomyelin (29.8 and 36.4%) on days 23 and 30 of embryo development, respectively.

Table 14.

Percentage content of individual phospholipid fractions in mitochondria of rabbit placenta at 30 days of pregnancy in normal and under the action of butifos (M + m,n=5-7).

Phospholipids	! Control !	Experience
Phosphatidylcholine	40,2+3,2	36,0+3,2
Phosphatidylethanolamine	15,1+1,1	9,4+0,9
Cardiolipin	5,0+0,4	13,2+0,8
Phosphatidylserine	5,7+0,2	2,7+0,2
Phosphatidylinositol	6,0+0,5	8,0+0,8
Sphingomyelin	8,5+0,5	11,6+0,7

Phosphatidic acid	I,8+0,3	I,2+0,1
Lys ophosphatidylcholine	4,0+0,4	0,9+0,01
Lysophosphatidylethanolamine	10,0+1,0	14,3+0,8
Lysocardiolipin	I,2+0,1	0,9+0,01
Lysophosphatidic acid	2,5+0,1	I,8+0,3

Analysis of absolute and relative changes in the content of lysocompounds under the action of butyphos to some extent explain the observed changes in the content of phospholipids. As our studies show, in mitochondria of placenta of experimental animals the content of lysophosphatidylcholine decreases sharply (by *76%)* and there is a tendency to increase the content of phosphatidylcholine. A similar picture is noted in the case of cardiolipin and lysocardiolipin. '

A marked decrease in the content of lysophosphatidylcholine and lysocardiolipin seems to be associated with the activation of endogenous lysophospholipases. The increase in cardiolipin content in placental mitochondria seems to be associated with an increase in the process of lipid synthesis. Kurysheva et al. (1974) showed that the placenta synthesises lipids independently. In contrast to lysophosphatidylcholine and lysocardiolipin, the content of lysophosphatidylethanolamine increased in placenta mitochondria (by 36.7 and 43.0%) with a simultaneous decrease in phosphatidylethanolamine, which suggests activation of phospholipase A_2 . It is interesting to note that under the action of butyphos both phosphatidic acid and lysophosphatidic acid are degraded at approximately the same rate. Apparently, in this case there is an inhibition of phosphatidic acid biosynthesis.

The ratio of phosphatidylcholine/phosphatidylethanolamine, in contrast to the similar index of fetal and maternal liver mitochondria, in placenta mitochondria increases by 1.26 and 1.44 times, respectively, at 23 and 30 days of embryo development (Fig.7, 8). These changes indicate deep disturbances in the placenta mitochondria membrane of experimental animals, since this ratio plays an important role for the functioning of membrane structures. We also found changes in the ratio of diacyl forms of phospholipids and their lysoforms. As a result of butifos action in placenta mitochondria, the phosphatidylcholine/lysophosphatidylcholine ratio increases 3.76 and 3.98 times, cardiolipin-lysocardiolipin - 3.16 and 3.53 times, and the phosphatidylethanolamine/lysophosphatidylethanolamine ratio decreases approximately 2-fold, respectively on days 23 and 30 of embryo development (Fig.7,8). Consequently, the effect of butyphos is characterised by changes in the ratio of lyso- and diacyl forms specific for each phospholipid form. Summarising the results obtained, it can be concluded that as a result of butifos action in placenta liver mitochondria the ratio of diacyl and lyso forms of phospholipids is disturbed, which in turn, apparently, leads to disturbance of mitochondrial functions and metabolism between mother and mitochondria and metabolism between mother and foetus.

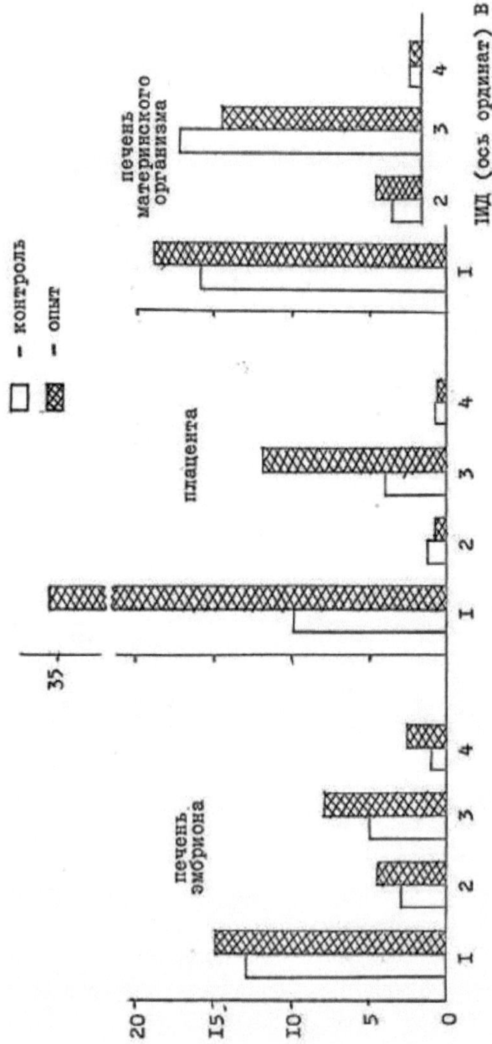

Figure 7. Influence of BUTIFOS on Phospholipid/Lysophosphos-Fo-Lipid Ratio (ordinate axis) in the MITOCHONDRY of Embryonic, Placenta and Rabbit Kidney at 23 days of gestation.
(I - FH/lFH ratio, 2 - PE/lFE, 3 - CL/lCL, 4- - FC/lFC)

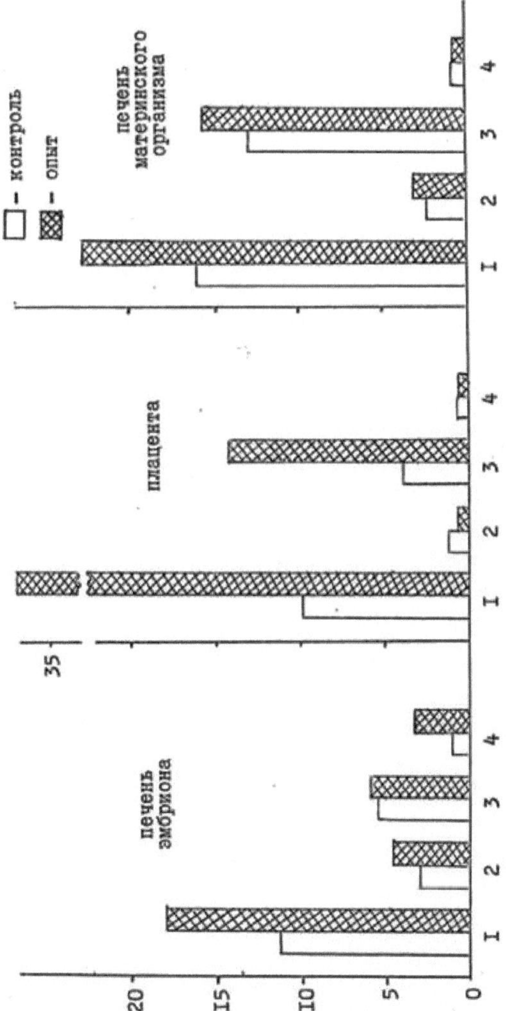

Figure 8. Influence of BUTIFOS on the F0SF0LIPID/Li30F0SF0LIPID ratio (ordinate axis) in the mitochondria of EMBRION, PLACENTA and rabbit livers at 30 days of gestation. (Both values are shown in Fig. 7)

Thus, a decrease in the content of lysophosphatidylcholines and lysocardiolipins is observed in mitochondria of the organs of animals studied by us under the action of butifos. At the same time, the content of other phospholipid fractions changes differently in response to butyphos action. For example, phosphatidylinositol levels are increased in maternal and placental liver mitochondria and decreased in fetal liver mitochondria. The content of lysophosphatidic acid is increased only in the mitochondria of the mother's liver, while in other cases, on the contrary, it is decreased.

It should be noted that under the influence of butyphos, the other phospholipid fractions change quantitatively in the same direction in fetal and maternal liver mitochondria compared to placental mitochondria. Thus, while the content of phosphatidylcholine, phosphatidylethanolamine, phosphatidylserine and phosphatidic acid in maternal and foetal liver mitochondria increases, the level of all these phospholipids in placental mitochondria decreases. At the same time, the content of cardiolipins, sphingomyelins and lysophosphatidylethanolamines changes in the opposite way. It should be noted that the most profound changes in the composition of phospholipids occur in the mitochondrial membrane of maternal and foetal liver mitochondria at later stages of development.

In mitochondria of the placenta of rabbits butifos-induced deviation of the content of some phospholipids from the normal level does not depend on the terms of embryo development. In general, changes in the content of phospholipids in mitochondria of the studied animal organs under the action of butyphos are obviously caused by disturbances in the synthesis of phospholipids in cell membranes and transport mechanisms from the endoplasmic reticulum to other membrane formations of the cell (Dyatlovitskaya et al., 1976; Bereziat, 1980), as well as by corresponding changes in the activity of endogenous phospholipases and lysophospholipases of mitochondria.

3.10. The effect of butifos on the protein composition of mitochondria of liver mitochondria of embryos, placenta and liver of pregnant rabbits.

It follows from the results of electrophoretic separation of mitochondrial proteins that after administration of butifos at a dose of 1/20 LD_{50} lipeptide-like fractions of liver mitochondria of 23- and 30-day embryos in the control and experiment give approximately the same electrophoretic and densitometric picture (Fig. 9, 10). The electrophoregram of proteins of mitochondria of placental mitochondria of rabbits at 30 days of gestation differs from the electrophoregram of proteins of mitochondria of 23-day placenta by a marked change in some protein fractions arising under the influence of butifos (Figs. II, 12). These changes are characterised by a decrease in fractions I-Sh and an increase in fraction 1U. In the electrophoregram of maternal liver mitochondria proteins we did not find any significant changes (data not presented).

Thus, butifos induces a change in the mitochondrial protein fractions of placental mitochondria of the fetal placenta. This change is probably related to the increased necessity of the role of the placenta in the realisation of its barrier function. Indeed, in the foetal period of development, the main organs of the foetus begin to function and the protective function of the placenta increases.

Figure 9. DENSITOGRAM OF MITOCHONDRIAL PROTEINS LIVERS OF 23-DAY-OLD EMBRYOS BY DISC ELECTROPHORESIS IN 11% PAATE IN THE PRESENCE OF *1%* SODIUM DODECYL SULFATE AND *1%* -MERCAPTOETHANOL.

A - control, B - experimental (when butifos was administered at a dose of 1/20 LD50).

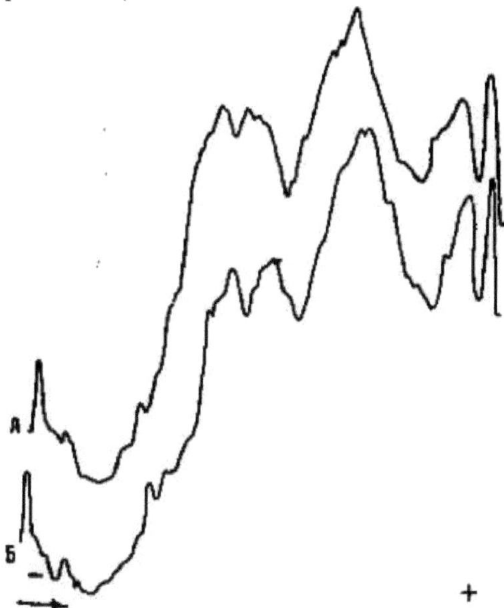

Figure 10. DENSITOGRAM OF LIVER MITOCHONDRIAL PROTEINS OF 30-DAY-OLD EMBRYOS BY DISC ELECTROPHORESIS IN 11% PAATE IN THE PRESENCE OF *1%* SODIUM DODECYL SULPHATE AND 1% - MERCAPTOETHANOL.

A - control, B - experimental (when butifos was administered at a dose of 1/20 LD50).

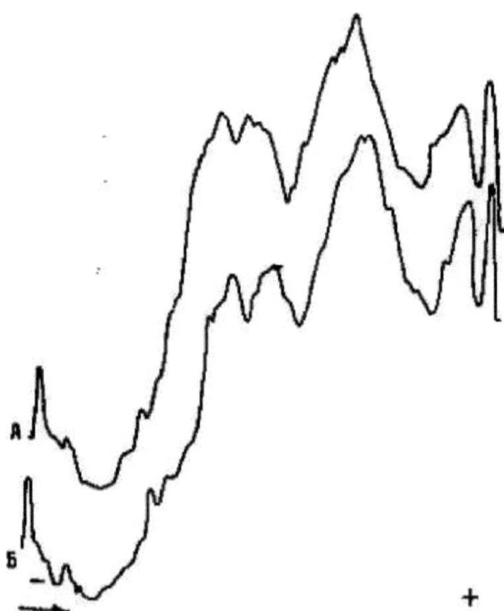

Fig. II. DENSITOGRAM OF PROTEINS OF MITOCHONDRIA OF RABBIT PLACENTA ON THE 23RD DAY OF PREGNANCY. DISC ELECTROPHORESIS IN 11% PAAG IN THE PRESENCE OF 1% SODIUM DODECYL SULFATE AND 1% MERCAPTOETHANOL.

A - control, B - experimental (when butifos was administered at a dose of 1/20 LD50).

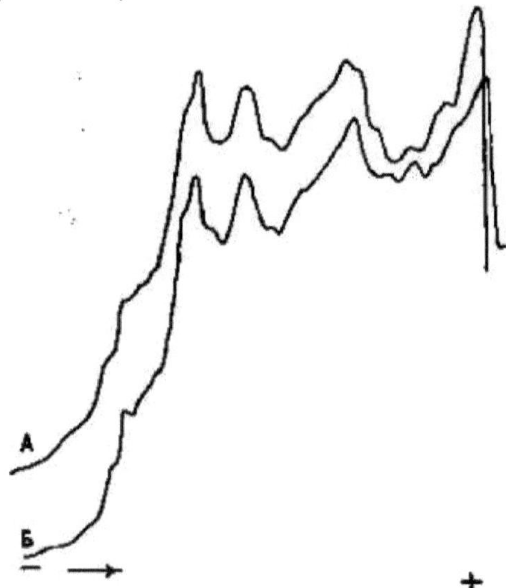

Figure 12. DENSITOGRAM OF PROTEINS OF MITOCHONDRIA OF RABBIT PLACENTA AT 30 DAYS OF PREGNANCY. DISC ELECTROPHORESIS IN 11% PAAG IN THE PRESENCE OF 1% SODIUM DODECYL SULFATE AND 1% -

MERCAPT03TAN0L.

A - control, B - experimental (when butifos was administered at a dose of 1/20 LD50).

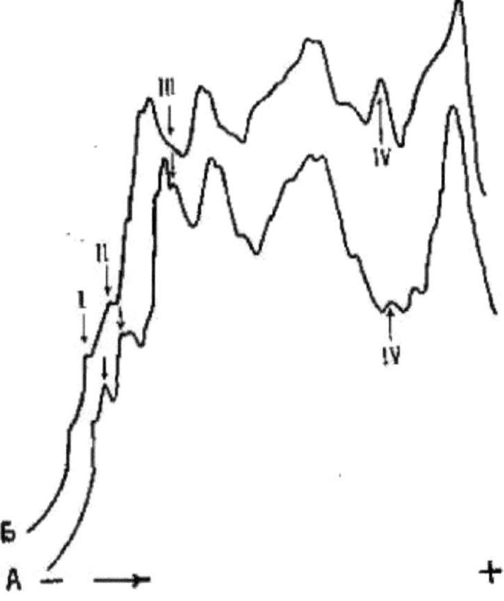

CONCLUSION

The study of abnormalities in fetal development under the influence of various pathogenic factors, including pesticides, is associated with the solution of the following problems: to study the condition of the maternal organism, to analyse the possibility of transplacental transfer of the damaging factor into the embryo organism and, finally, to study the development and condition of the embryo. To evaluate the effect of butifos on the mother-placenta-fetus complex, we used mitochondria as a test system. It is known that these intracellular organelles are the most sensitive part of the cell, and their reactions and state determine the reactions and state of the whole cell (Skulachev, 1962; Kondrashova, 1968). It is also well known that phospholipids are an essential constituent of biological membranes. They play an important structural and functional role in maintaining the constancy of physicochemical characteristics of the cytosol and other compartments, in the regulation of the functions of membrane formations and the activity of membrane-bound enzymes. On this basis, we investigated changes in the phospholipid composition of mitochondrial membranes of maternal liver and placenta and foetal liver mitochondria in normal and under the influence of butyphos.

To compare the directionality of changes in some parameters characterising functional activity or structural role in mitochondrial membranes, they are shown in Table 15, where changes in the experiment (butyphos) versus control are estimated in semi-quantitative terms. Indeed, inoculation of animals with butyphos leads to certain changes in functions, activity of membrane-bound enzymes and phospholipid spectrum in mitochondria of the studied animal organs (Table 15). For example, in mitochondria of liver of the maternal organism there is a decrease of con-

Table 15.

Summary table of changes in various parameters studied induced in embryo and maternal liver mitochondria and in placenta mitochondria under the influence of butyphos administration.

(Changes are given relative to control. + - increase in value parameter; 2 - decrease; o - no change)

Mitochondria parameter under study	23 days			30 days		
	Ebrio liver	Placenta	Liver mothers	Ebrio liver	Ebrio liver	Liver mothers
1	2	3	4	5	6	7
1. oxidative phosphorylation (substrate succinate)						
V4*	0	++	-	-	-	0

V4	+	++	-	0	-	0
V3	++	-	0	-	-	-
V3p	+++	+	0	-	-	0
DK	+	-	+	-	+++	-
ADP/O	+	-	+	-	0	+
Substrate-glutamate						
V4 *	0		-	-		-
V4	-		-	-		-
V3	+		+	-		-
Vip	+		-	-		-
DK	++		+	-		0
ADP/O	+		+	0		+
2. Succinate oxidase	++	-	-	++	-	-
3. Cytochrome c-oxidase	+	-	-	++	-	-
1	2	3	4	5	6	7
4.NAD.H- oxidase general.	+	-	-	+	-	-
Same + cytochrome c	++	-	-	+	-	-
Rotenone- insensitive	++	-	-	++	-	-
Rothenon-sensitive	-	-	-	-	-	-
5. Phospholipid composition						
Phosphotidylchol n	+	+	+	+	+	+
Phophotidylethanol amine	+	-	+	+	-	+
Cardiolipin	+	+++	-	++	+++	-
Phosphotidylserine	+++	-	++	+++	-	++
Phosphotidylinositol	-	++	0	-	++	+++
Sphingomyelin	++	++	-	+++	++	-
Phosphotidic acid	+	-	+	++	-	++
Lysophosphotidylch OLIN	-	-	-	-	-	-
Lysophosphatidylene tanolamine	-	++	-	-	+++	-
Lysocardiolipin	-	-	-	-	-	-
Lysophosphatidic acid	-	-	+	-	-	+
FH/LFH	+	+++	+	+++	+++	+++
PE/IFE	++	-	++	+++	-	+++
KL/LKL	+++	+++	-	0	+++	++
FC/LFC	+++	-	0	+++	0	+
Protein composition	0	0	0	0	-	0

cardiolipin, sphingomyelin, lysophosphatidylcholine, lyso- phosphatidylethanolamine and lysocardiolipin with simultaneous increase in the content of phosphatidylcholine, phosphatidylethanolamine, phosphatidylinositol, phosphatidylserine, phosphatidic acid and its lysosoe- dination.

Butiphos in placenta mitochondria leads to a decrease in the content of phosphatidylethanolamine, phosphatidylserine, phosphatidylcholine and its lysocompounds, lysocardiolipin, phosphatidic acid and its lysocompounds, and an increase in cardiolipin, phosphatidylinositol, sphingomyelin and lysophosphatidylethanolamine. At the same time in mitochondria of embryo liver under the influence of butifos there is a decrease in the level of cardiolipin, phosphatidylinositol, sphingomyelin and all fractions of lysophospholipids. At the same time, an increase in the content of phosphatidylcholine , phosphatidylethanolamine, phosphatidylserine and phosphatidic acid was observed. It should be noted that butyphos-induced changes in the content of phospholipids and their lysocompounds in mitochondria of liver, maternal placenta and foetal liver increase most significantly at 30 days of embryonic development.

The results of the study of respiration, oxidative phosphorylation and activity of polyenzyme systems of mitochondrial membranes of the studied organs during this period of pregnancy also differ most significantly in the experiment and control. For example, at early terms of embryo development (23 days) the effect of butifos is characterised by a decrease in the rate of succinate oxidation in maternal liver mitochondria in V_4 *HV_4 , proceeding without significant changes in the rate of phosphorylation and DNF-stimulated oxidation. On the contrary, the rate of glutamate oxidation in the V_4 *H V_4 state does not change, while the rate of phosphorylation and DNF-stimulated oxidation increases to some extent.

However, the conjugation of mitochondrial preparations (see DC and ADP/0) at this term under the influence of butyphos is increased in media with both oxidation substrates. At 30 days of embryonic development, only the rate of phosphorylation-dependent succinate oxidation is decreased without significant changes in other mitochondrial metabolic states. However, the rate of glutamate oxidation decreases and the ADP/0 ratio increases to some extent in media with both oxidation substrates.

Mitochondria isolated from the placenta of experimental rabbits were characterised by accelerated respiration at early embryonic development (23 days) and suppression of mitochondrial respiratory function at 30 days of development. While in the former case (23 days) the efficiency of oxidative phosphorylation (ADP/0,DA) decreased, in contrast, in the latter case it increased to some extent. Other patterns are revealed in the case of embryonic liver mitochondria. On the 23rd day of eebrio development in foetal liver mitochondria, an acceleration of respiration and efficiency of oxidative phosphorylation is observed, while on the 30th day, on the contrary, the rate of electron transfer and the activity of the energy conversion system are suppressed.

In the model we used, we studied the relatively distant (10-day period) biochemical consequences of treating animals with mild doses (1/20 LD_{50}) of butifos. It is clear that under these conditions direct effects of the studied pesticide on mitochondrial functions can be excluded, and the measured parameters of their functional state obviously reflect changes in the number of respiratory transporters and (or) activity of the systems of transport of respiratory and phosphorylation substrates through the inner membrane of mitochondria. Modification of the lipid microenvironment of membrane-bound enzymes may play an important functional role in these conditions.

In general, the changes in the parameters of oxidative phosphorylation of mitochondria of placenta, maternal liver and embryo induced by low doses of butyphos have, apparently, compensatory and tissue-specific character. Changes in the activity of the oxidative phosphorylation process are the most intensive on the 30th day in the mitochondria of the liver of embryos and placenta compared to the mitochondria of the mother's liver. This indicates the embryotropic effect of low doses of butifos, which undoubtedly has a complex nature including modification of mitochondrial functions.

Changes in the respiration rate of intact mitochondria can be caused not only by changes in the number of respiratory transporters in the electron transport chain or by selective blocking of the latter, but also by the influence of the microenvironment of respiratory chain components and the activity of substrate transport systems across the inner mitochondrial membrane. That is why we studied the activity of oxidase systems under conditions excluding the limit at the stage of substrate transport.

The study of the state of oxidase systems of mitochondria membranes of the studied organs shows that butifos hpuhuo leads to a decrease in the activity of succinatoxidase and cytochrome c-oxidase systems of the respiratory chain of mitochondria of placenta and liver of the maternal organism, but increases their activity in mitochondria of the liver of embryos. When analysing the ratio of NAD.H oxidation rates by internal and external oxidation pathways, it can be seen that the activity of both systems of mitochondria of both liver and placenta of the maternal organism decreases under the influence of butifos. The activity of rotenone-sensitive NAD.H-oxidase system decreases especially markedly. In embryo liver mitochondria, the activity of both systems increases, and the activity of the rotenone-insensitive pathway of NAD.H oxidation is especially marked.

The data characterising the level of activity of polyenzyme systems together with the characterisation of parameters of oxidative phosphorylation of mitochondria testify to the tissue-specific and embryotropic effect of low doses of butifos. Indeed, in both cases, the most noticeable changes under the influence of the pesticide were observed in the parameters related to mitochondria of embryo liver - on 30 days of development there was a dissociation of oxidative phosphorylation, some inhibition of respiration, despite the above described increase in the activity of oxidase systems.

The study of the effect of exogenous cytochrome c on the rate of NAD.H oxidation in norm and during butifos administration to animals showed that the pesticide leads to an increase in the activity of rotenone-insensitive NAD.H-oxidase and a decrease in the activity of rotenone-sensitive NAD.H-oxidase system of the mitochondrial respiratory chain. Absolute values of NAD.H-oxidase activity both in the presence and absence of exogenous cytochrome c are highest in embryonic liver mitochondria, and maternal administration of low doses of butifos induces an additional increase in oxidase activity in its rotenone-sensitive (internal pathway) and rotenone-insensitive (external pathway) branches. In the case of maternal liver mitochondria and placental mitochondria, such induction is absent.

Under the conditions used to determine the activity of polyenzyme systems, the maximum rate of electron transfer along the respiratory chain or its segments is detected, and the respiration rate of intact isolated mitochondria may be only a part of the oxidase activity. However, information on the potential activity of the respiratory system is important for assessing the diverse role of mitochondria under physiological conditions, which is to supply "building material" for plastic metabolism, especially in developing tissues and organs, in heat reduction, detoxification, etc. (Skulachev, 1969). In this connection, the observed increase in the activity of oxidase systems in the mitochondria of the embryo liver seems to be natural, indicating the intensification under the influence of butifos of a number of metabolic processes in the embryo liver, which are registered by the rate of electron transfer along the respiratory chain.

Thus, butyphos induces changes in the content of major and minor fractions of phospholipids in the mitochondrial membrane of the studied animal organs. As a result of these and, apparently, some other changes, respiration, oxidative phosphorylation and activity of polyenzyme systems of mitochondrial membranes are disturbed. The accessibility of exogenous cytochrome c to the corresponding regions of the inner membrane of mitochondria of the studied animal organs is also modified. The most profound structural and functional changes under the influence of butyphos are observed at late terms of embryonic development.

conclusions

1 When butifos was administered to rabbits at a dose of 1/20 LD_{50} on day 23 of gestation, a decrease in the rate of succinate oxidation (by 20%) by maternal liver mitochondria was observed, while the rate of ADP- and DNF-stimulated respiration did not differ from the control.

2 As a result of butifos administration, the rate of succinate oxidation increased in all metabolic states, most significantly in the state (placenta mitochondria) and (embryo liver mitochondria). In media with glutamate under the influence of butyphos, similar changes were observed.

3 Butifos administration induces on the 30th day of pregnancy a general inhibition of mitochondrial respiration, especially expressed in the metabolic state V_3 (mitochondria of maternal and foetal liver) and V4 (mitochondria of placenta and foetal liver).

4 Under the influence of butifos, changes in the activity of oxidase systems and disruption of the access of exogenous cytochrome c to the corresponding parts of mitochondrial membranes were observed. The activity of NAD.H-oxidase, succinatoxidase and cytochrome c-oxidase in the mitochondria of the foetal liver increases in all periods, while in the mitochondria of the placenta and maternal body, on the contrary, it decreases markedly.

5 Under the influence of butifos, the activity of rotenone-insensitive NAD.H-oxidase system of embryo liver mitochondria is mainly increased and, on the contrary, the activity of rotenone-sensitive NAD.H-oxidase system of placenta and maternal liver mitochondria is inhibited.

6 Butifos administration induces changes in the content of some major and minor components of phospholipid fractions of mitochondria of embryo liver, maternal organism, and placenta, which are most pronounced by 30 days of embryonic development and correlate with the parameters of the functional state of mitochondria. The ratio of protein fractions of mitochondria, according to the data of analytical disc electrophoresis in PAGE, practically does not change in all studied preparations, except for mitochondria of placenta of 30-day embryos.

REFERENCE LIST

1. Agzamov X., Almatov K.T., Gulyamov T.D., Rakhimov M.M. Activity and stability of polyenzyme systems of liver mitochondrial membranes in chronic allergic ulcerative colitis. - Voprosy med.chemii, 1981, vol. 27, vol. 5, p. 658-662.
2. Agzamov X., Almatov K.T., Rakhimov M.M., Turakulov Y.H., Functioning of liver mitochondria in alloxan diabetes. - Voprosy med.chemii, 1983, vol. 29, vol. I, pp. 61-66.
3. Agureev A.P., Altukhov N.D., Mokhova E.N., Savelyev I.A. Activation of external oxidation of NAD.H in mitochondria at decreasing pH. - Biochemistry, 1981, vol. 46, vol. II, pp. 1945-1956.
4. Akberov R.S. Oxidative phosphorylation of mitochondria of rabbit placenta at poisoning by chlorophos and phosphacol. - In the book: "Republican n.-technical conf. on problems of veterinary medicine. Tez.dokl., Kazan, 1978, p. 22-23.
5. Almatov K.T., Agzamov X., Rakhimov M.M., Turakulov Y.H. Quantitative assessment of hidden damage in mitochondrial membranes. - Uzbek Biol. Zhurnal, 1981, No. 2, pp. 3-7.
6. Almatov K.T. Gulyamov T.D. Functional state of mitochondria of pancreas at introduction of chlorophos and hekeachloro-cyclohexane. - In the book: "Theses of Dokl. 3 conf. of biochemists of Central Asia and Kazakhstan. Dushanbe: Donish, 1981, p. 198.
7. Almatov K.T., Agzamov X., Rakhimov M.M. Oxidative phosphorylation in mitochondria of digestive organs in chronic allergic colitis. - Voprosy med.chemii, 1982, vol.28,
. vol. I, pp. 44-49.
8. Andrashko V.V., Levanyuk V.F., Kamoso M.A., Hryzhak
I.P. Effect of chlorophos on energy metabolism in placenta and organs of intrauterine foetus. - Pharmacol. and Toxicol. 1975, Vol. 38, No. 2,
c.208-209.
9. Anina I.A. The possibility of using the indicators of nucleic acid metabolism for predicting the remote effects of some pesticides. - Hygiene of labour and occupational diseases, M.: Medicine, 1975, No.1, pp.51-53.
10. Archakov A.I. Molecular organisation and function of electron transfer chains of membranes of the endoplasmic reticulum of the liver. - Uspekhi sovrem, Biol., 1971, vol. 71, vol. 2, p.163-183.
11. Akhmadjanov K. Correlation of some indicators of peripheral blood under the influence of organophosphorus compounds of low intensity in experiment. - In the book: "Actual issues of pesticide application in different climatic-geographical zones. Yerevan: Hayastan, 1976, p.129-131.
12. Akhmerova A. A. Histological changes in the organs of experimental animals under the influence of some pesticides. - In collection: Materials of the republican scientific-practical conf. on hygiene problems in conditions of Uzbekistan. Tashkent, 1970, p.287-290.

13. Akhmerova A.A., Babadjanova M.S., Melnikova E.V. Histological changes in the organs of experimental animals under the influence of some chemicals. - In Collected Works: Problems of Hygiene and Health Care Organisation in Uzbekistan. Tashkent, 1976, issue 3, p.151-153.
14. Badaeva L.N., Kisileva N.I., Pismennaya M.B. Morphology
Neurotoxicity of some organochlorine and organophosphorus pesticides in the mother-fetus system. In the book: Hygiene of application, toxicology
Pesticides and clinic of poisoning. M.: Medicine, 1981, № 12, p.106109.
15. Barilyak I.R., Kalinovskaya L.P. Ultrastructure of embryonic hepatocyte under chloridine action in conditions of blockade of synthesis
16. RNA. - Cytology and Genetics, 1977, vol. I, no. 3, pp. 213-217.
16. Barilyak J.R., Kalinovskaya L.P. Histochemical and ultrastructural characteristics of embryonic hepatocyte under the action of chloridine (pyrimethamine). - Cytology and Genetics, 1979, vol.
XSH, no. 2, pp. 83-92.
17. Bergelson L.D. - Biological membranes. Facts and hypotheses. - M.: Nauka, 1975, - 184 pp.
18. Besschetnikov I.I., Chorayan O.G. Dynamics of information characteristics of the chemical composition of developing organs of chicken embryos. - Archives of Anatomy, Histology and Embryology, 1981, vol. II, No. I, pp. 89-92.
19. Birchmeier W. Structure of cytochrome c-oxidase from baker's pecans
yeast. - Molecular genetics of mitochondria. L.: Nauka, 1977,
c. 133-138.
20. Borovyagin V. L. On the interpretation of data of electron microscopy methods in the study of structural organisation of model and biological membranes. - In Vn.: Biophysics (Results of Science and Technology), vol. 4 (methods of studying the structure of biological membranes). Moscow: VINITI, 1974, pp. 226-287.
21. Weber R. Electron-microscopic study of embryonic differentiation. - In: Ultrastructure and Function of the Cell. M.: Mir, 1965, pp. 225-233.
22. Verzhbinskaya N.A.Oxidative phosphorylation in the brain
of vertebrates at different stages of ontogenesis. In: U International Biochem. congress. Symp. 5: Intracellular respiration:
Phosphorylating and non-phosphorylating oxidation reactions. M.: Nauka, 1961, pp. 14-20.
23. Vinogradov A.D. Succinate dehydrogenase: structure and functions. Author's thesis, M., 1982, - 32 p.
24. Voronina V.M. Experimental data on the embrmotoxic effect of phthalophos. - In: Hygiene of application, toxicology of pesticides and clinic of poisoning. Kiev: VNshGmNTOKS, 1971, p. 254-257.
25. Gavrikova E.V., Goloveshkina V.G., Vinogradov A.D. New catalytic centre of succinate dehydrogenase. - In the book: Mitochondria. Energy Accumulation and Regulation of Enzymatic Processes. Moscow: Nauka, 1977, p.123-129.

26. Hofmekler V.A., Khuriev B.B., Danilov V.D. Effect of small concentrations of methylmercaptophos on the fecundity of female white rats.
In Collection: Mater, scientific-practical conf. of the Resp. society of pathologists of Uzbekistan. Tashkent: Medicine, 1969, p.53-55.
27. Gofmekler V.A., Khuriev B.B., Danilov V.D. Abnormalities of embryo development during inhalation exposure of pregnant white rats to methylmercaptophos. Ibid, pp.56-58.
28. Gofmekler V.A., Tabakova S.A. Effect of chlorophos on rat embryogenesis. - Pharmacol. and Toxicol., M., 1970, Vol. 33, No. 6, p.735737.
29. Gofmekler V.A., Khuriev B.B. Experimental study of embryonic action of methylmercaptophos at inhalation intake into the organism. - Hygiene and Sanitation, 1971, No.1, p.27-32.
30. Gofmekler V. A. Embriotropic effect of chemical pollutants of atmospheric air. - Hygiene and Sanitation, 1974, No. 9,
c. 7-10.
31. Green D.E., Fleischer S. Molecular organisation of biological transforming systems. - In: Horizons of Biochemistry. M.: Mir, 1964, pp.293-325.
31. Green D.E., Goldberger R. - Molecular aspects of life. -
M.: Mir. 1968,c.
32. Gulyamov T.D., Almatov K.T. Effect of hexachlorocyclohexane and chlorophos on oxidative phosphorylation and activity of polyenzyme systems of pancreatic mitochondrial membranes.
- Manuscript deposited in VINITI on 5 Oct. 1981 № 4685.81 - Dei. USSR ACADEMY OF MEDICAL SCIENCES. M.: VINITI, 1981, p.9.
1974, Jamalutdinov R. Influence of some pesticides on protein composition of blood serum in animals. In the book: Actual problems of modern medicine. Mater, nauk. conf. Tashkent: Medicine, part 1, p. 1. 68-69.
33. Dzhurayeva M.M. Phospholipids of nuclear and mitochondrial phospholipids
Membranes under irradiation during embryonic development. - Cand. diss. Biol. of Sciences, Tashkent, 1983, - 107 pp.
34. Dolgo-Saburov V.B. Activity of some enzymes and
tissue and serum isoenzymes in seizure states.
In book: 2nd VBS. Theses of sectional reports. Tashkent: Fan, 1969, Section 21, p.30.
35. Dolgo-Saburov V.B., Palkanova M.S. Action of chlorophos on the
mitochondrial membranes of white rat liver. - Pharmacol. and Toxicol, 1982, No. 4, pp. 67-70.
36. Dyban A.P., Akimova I.M., Svetlova V.A. Effect of 2,4-diamino-5-chlorophenyl-6-ethylpyrimidine on the embryonic development of rats.Dokl. ANSSR, 1965, Vol. 163, No. 6, pp. I5I4-I5I8.
37. Dyatlovitskaya E.V., Timofeeva N.G., Grkova N.P., Bereglson
Л. D. Phospholipid exchange between mitochondria and microsomes of rat hepatoma 27. - Biochemistry, 1976, vol. 41, issue 7, pp. 1235-1240. and40. Dyatlovitskaya E.V.,

Sinitsina E.V., Timofeeva N.G., Kuprina N.I., Ridinskaya T.D., Bergelson L.D. Immunological detection of sphingomyelin transfer protein in tumours and embryonic liver of rats. - Biochemistry, 1982, Vol. 47, No. I, pp. 62-65.
38. Evtodienko Y.V., Medvedev B.I., Kudzina L.Y., Kobelev B.C., Yaguzhinsky L.S., Kuzin A.M. Identification of a compound inducing transport of potassium ions in mitochondria and bilayer membranes. - Dokl. of the USSR Academy of Sciences, 1977, vol. 233, *Sh* 4, p. 708-711.
39. Zhdanovich N.V., Udalev Y.F. Role of vitamin and pyridoxine
in FOS intoxication. - Military Medical Journal, 1969, No. 8, pp. 58-61.
40. Zabusov B.G. Histochemical and pathomorphological study of acute lethal poisoning by some FOS in experiment.
41. In book: Histochemistry in normal and pathological morphology. Novosibirsk, 1967, pp. 358-360.
42. Zagoruiko G.V., Peskareva E.V., Mahinko V.I.
Electron-microscopic structure of liver parenchyma cells in embryogenesis of the domestic duck. - In Book: Molecular and physiol. mechanisms of age development. Kiev: Naukova Dumka, 1975, p. 346354.
43. Zainutdinov B.R., Sadykov S., Shulakova T.Y., Isaev E.I. Phospholipids of heart and liver mitochondria during embryogenesis. In Vn.: Biochemistry of mitochondria. Moscow: Nauka, 1976, p. 166.
44. Zakirov U.B., Kadyrov U.Z., Volokhviansky E.A. Influence of butifos on enzyme-forming function of small intestine. - Toxicol. and Pharmacol. 1975, No. I, pp. 96-99.
45. Zybina E.V. Ultrastructure of the rabbit oocyte at the stage of bilayer follicle. - Cytology, 1975, Vol. 18, N° 2, p. 126-129.
46. Ivanova T.M., Dolgo-Saburov V.B., Stroikov Y.N. Changes in the energy function of mitochondria under the action of eserine and pi-crotoxin. - Ukr. biochemical journal, 1978, vol. 50, no. 6, pp. 691- 694.
47. Kagan Y.S. Actual questions of hygiene and toxicology. D
Collection: Hygiene of application, toxicology of pesticides and clinic of poisoning. 1970, vol. 8, p. 18-30.
48. Kagan Y.S., Sasinovich L.M., Voronina L.Ya. On the chronic effect of some pesticides on the functional state of the liver. - Hygiene and Sanitation, 1970, No. 9, p. 36-39.
49. Kagan Y.S. Actual issues of toxicological study of pesticides. - In Vn.: Plant Protection. Moscow: VINITI, 1972, vol. I, p. 285-330.
50. Kadyrov U.Z., Zakirov U.B., Volokhoviansky E.A. Enzymatic activity of small intestine in acute butifos poisoning. - Med.zhurnal Uzbekistana, 1982, № 6, p. 46-48.
51. Kaloyanova F., Ivanova L., Dimov G., Mukhtarova M. Experimental substantiation of maximum permissible concentration of BI-58 in atmospheric air. - Hygiene and Sanitation, 1968, No.6, p.**6-10**.
52. Campo M.A. Effect of chlorophos on oxygen uptake in the placenta of rabbits. - Ukr. biochem. journal, 1982, vol. 54, No. 4, p. 455- 457.

53. Campo M.A. Redox processes in the placenta during pregnancy failure and experimental exposure to some biochemically active substances. - Avtoref. kand. diss.. Biol. of Sciences, Lvov, 1983, 17 p.
54. Kargapolov A.V., Kartseva S.V. Method of simultaneous fractionation of the main fractions of lysophospholipids and their diacyl derivatives. - Voprosy med.chemii, 1975, vol. 21, pp. 325-327.
55. Kargapolov A.V., Kartseva S.V., Semenova E.G., Mikelsaar X.0 phospholipid composition of adenosine triphosphatase complex from bovine heart mitochondria. - Sci. dokl. higher school. Biol.nauki, 1975, vol. 2, p. 50-55.
56. Kargapolov A.V. Changes in the phospholipid composition of intact mitochondria during their swelling in hypotonic sucrose solution. - Biochemistry, 1979, vol. 44, issue 2, p.293-296.
57. KargapolovA. V. Lipid composition analysis mitochondrial and endoplasmic membranes using the method of of horizontal flow chromatography. -Biochemistry , 1981, t 46,vol.4,pp.691-698.
58. Karmilov V.A. Subacute experimental poisoning by chlorophos. - Pharmacol. and Toxicol. 1973, No.6, p.727-728.
59. Karmilov V. A. Activity of succinate dehydrogenase and of tissue cytochrome oxidase in chlorophos intoxication. - In Book: Problems of Pathology in Experiment and Clinic. Moscow: Medicine, 1974, vol. 1, p. 266-268.
60. KasymovaR .A. Experimental study of the embryotoxic effect of butifos. - Uzbek Biol.Zhurnal, 1975, No.4, p.30-32.
61. Knysh B.C. Separate and combined effect of some organophosphorus pesticides on organism. - Cand. diss. Biol. of Sciences, Alma-Ata, 1980, - p. p.
62. Knyazeva JI.C., Najmutdinov K.N., Hakimov 3.3. Effect of butifos on some histochemical and biochemical indices of the liver of white rats. - Pharmacol. and toxicol. Tashkent, 1975. p. p. 105-108.
63. Kovalenok A.V., Kazanova T.P. Change of activity level Succinate dehydrogenase in the housefly during chlorophos and gamma-hexachlorane poisoning. - Izvestiya SO AS USSR, ser.biol.Novosibirsk, 1967, № 2, p. II8-I22.
64. Koval T.Yu. Effect of thyroxine on the energy metabolism of mitochondria of developing tissues. - Abstract of Cand. diss.... Biol. of Sciences, Tashkent, 1979, - 19 p.
65. Kondrashova M.N. Biochemical excitation cycle. - In the book: Mitochondria. Enzymatic processes and their regulation. Moscow: Nauka, 1968, c. I22-131*
66. Kondrashova M.N. Regulation by succinic acid of energy supply and functional state of tissue. - Author's abstract of doctoral dissertation. Biol. sciences, Pushchino, 1971, - 52 pp.
67. Konstantinov Y.M., Filippova S.N., Vavilin V.A., Panov A.V., Lyakhovich V.V.. Changes in oxidative phosphorylation in rat liver mitochondria during the

development of cholestasis. - Voprosy med.chemii, 1980, vol. 26, No. 4, pp. 498-501.
69. Crepe E.M. - Lipids of cell membranes. - L.: Nauka, 1981, - 339 pp.
70. Kundiev Y.I. Absorption of pesticides through the skin and prevention of poisoning. - Kiev: Zdorovye, 1975, - 200 pp.
71. Kur. D.A., Iskandarov T.P. Some biochemical shifts in the combined effect of gamma-isomer HCGC and methyl mercaptophos. - In the book: Mater. Sh congress of hygienists, sanitary doctors, epidemiologists, microbiologists and infectious diseases specialists of Uzbekistan. Tashkent: Medicine, 1973, p. II6-II7.
72. Kur D.A. Biological effect of organophosphorus pesticides depending on their chemical structure. - Med.zhurnal Uzbekistana, 1974, No. 2, pp. 3-6.
73. Kurambaev Y.K. Influence of small doses of organophosphorus pesticide antio on secretion and ratio of glucocorticoid hormones of adrenal cortex. - In the book: Actual issues of immunol. and toxicol. Theses of reports of the 5th Resp. conf. of the Central Scientific Research Centre of Medical Universities of Uzbekistan. 1981, Tashkent, p. 113-114.
74. Kurysheva K. A., Stolnikova I.I., Kolgushkin G. G. A., Goncharova V. G. Features of lipid composition of blood serum of mother, newborn and placenta during physiological course of pregnancy and labour. - Obstetrics and Gynaecol. 1983, No. 3, pp. 6-9.
75. Levskaya E.N. Methylmercaptophos. Plenum on the results of State tests of pesticides and biopreparations in 1973.
76. Leibovich D.L. Evaluation of embryotropic action of low doses Organophosphorus pesticides - chlorophos, metaphos and Carbophos.Hygiene and Sanitation, 1973, No. I, pp. 21-24.
77. Leninger A.L. - Mitochondria. - M.: Mir, 1966, p.- 316.
78. Leninger A.L. - Biochemistry. - M.: Mir, - 1974, - 957 pp.
79. .Martson L.V., Voronina V.M. Experimental study of the Effect of organophosphorus pesticides dipterex and imidan on embryogenesis. - In the book: Mater. I final Soviet-American Symp. on the problem: "Environmental Hygiene", Riga, 1974.M.: Medicine, 1975, p. 163-172.
80. MakhinkoV .I., ShchegolkovV .N. Oxidative Phosphorylation of mitochondria in the liver of duck embryos during the second half of development. - In the book: Problems of Age Physiol., Biochem. and Biophys. Kiev: Naukova Dumka, 1974, p. 231-236.
81. Medved L.I., Kagan Y.S., Spinu E.I. Pesticides and public health problems. - Journal of the D.I. Mendeleev WHO, 1968, No. 3, pp. 263-271.
82. Medved L.I. - Reference book on pesticides. - Kiev: Urozhay, 1977, - 265 pp.
83. Melnikov N.N. Journal of the D.I. Mendeleev WHO, 1973, vol. 18, No. 5, p. 482.
84. Mirahmedov A.K., Sheraliev A., Almatov K.T., Khamidov D.H. Effect of butifos on respiration and oxidative phosphorylation of liver mitochondria of embryos and pregnant rabbits. - Uzbek Biol.Zhurnal, 1984, No.2, p.50-52.
85. Mikelsaar X., Severina I.M., Skulachev V.P. Phospholipids and oxidative

phosphorylation. - Uchpekhisovrem ,
Biol.,1974,vol.3(6), pp. 348-370.
86. Musaev H.N., Almatov K.T., Rakhimov M.M., Akhmedov R.. Functioning of mitochondria of the small intestine mucosa under the influence of high temperature on the rat organism. - Voprosy med.chemii, 1981, vol. 27, vol. 6, p.763-768.
87. Najmutdinov K.N., Murzabekov S.M., Knyazeva L.S. Influence of pesticides on the general morphology and some histochemical indices of rat liver. - In Vb.: Voprosy pharmakol. i toxikol., Tashkent, 1975, p.103-108.
88. Novitskaya G.V. - Methodical guide on thin-layer chromatography of phospholipids. - Moscow: Nauka, 1972, - 103 pp.
1978, Ozernyuk N.D. Growth and reproduction of mitochondria. M.,Nauka,p.263.
89. Panov A .V., Lyakhovich V.V. Mitochondrial
adenine nucleotide-tra- nslokase. - Bioorganic Chemistry, 1978, Vol. 4, No. I, p.518.
90. Panov A.V., Vavilin V. A. A., Soloviev A.A., Lyakhovich V.V.. Relationship between the adenine nucleotide system and oxidative phosphorylation in rat liver in the dynamics of starvation. - Biochemistry, 1983, vol. 48, vol. 2, p.235-243.
91. Panshina T.N. Changes in conditioned-reflex activity and blood cholinesterase activity under the influence of organophosphorus insecticide phosphamide. - Bull. exp. biol. and med. 1963, № 12, p.56-60.
92. Patrikeeva M.V. Phospholipids of mitochondria of nervous system in ontogenesis of chickens. - Dokl. of the USSR Academy of Sciences, 1964, v.154, p.1235-1237.
93. Poglazov A.F. Investigation of physicochemical properties of mitochondrial outer membranes. - Cand. diss. Biol. of Sciences, M., 1973, - 136 pp.
94. Rodionov G.A., Voronina L.Y. Influence of chlorophos on development and course of liver pathology in experiment. - Physician's Business, 1973, No. II, pp. 51-58.
95. Rodionov G. A. To the problem of studying the pathogenic influence of chemical substances of the external environment on the organism. - Archiv, Pathol. v. 10, p. 48-52.
96. Rakhimov M.M. Almatov K.T. Some features of degradation of polyenzyme systems of rat liver mitochondria exposed to heat. - Biochemistry, 1977, vol. 42, vol. 10, pp. I852-1863.
97. Rakhimov M.M., Almatov K.T. Influence of calcium ions on the interaction of phospholipase D with phospholipids of mitochondrial membranes. - Biochemistry, 1978, vol. 43, issue 8, pp. 1390-1403.
98. Rotenberg Yu.S. Problem of influence of industrial toxic substances on bioenergetic processes of an organism in hygiene and toxicology. - Avtoref. dokt. diss.. Biol. sciences, M., 1980,. - 50 c.
99. Rybalchenko V.K., Kurskiy M.D. Role of lipids in biological membranes. Molecular organisation and enzymatic activity of biological membranes. - Kiev: Naukova Dumka, 1977, -210 p.
100. Racker E. - Bioenergetic Mechanisms. New views. - M.:. Mir, 1979, - 216 p.

101. Saidkasymova N.M., Ablyaeva N.H. Characteristics of energy disturbances in liver cells under exposure to bazudine. - Collected in: Problems of hygiene and toxicology of pesticides, Kiev: Nauko va dumka, 1981, part P, p. P., p. 142. 142.
102. Sayramanova Z.S. Influence of some pesticides on the generative function of animals. - In the collection: Actual problems of obstetrics and gynaecology. Tashkent: Medicine, 1971, p. 3-21.
103. Sentyurova L.G. Histogenesis of the liver and dynamics of the content in the of copper, zinc, iron and some oxidoreductases in pre- and postnatal ontogenesis of the rabbit. - Avtoref. kand. diss. of biology. sciences, Astrakhan, 1975, - 21 p.
104. Simonyan A. A. On the influence of lipoprotein fraction isolated from the liver of chicken embryo on oxidative phosphorylation. - In the book: Mitochondria. Biological functions in the system of cell organelles. Moscow: Nauka, 1969, pp. II6-II9.
105. Simonyan A.A., Abramyan K.S., Gevorkyan G.A., Bodlyan R.B., Shatrerova A.A. Ultrastructural changes in mitochondria of chicken heart and liver in ontogenesis. - Biol. journal of Armenia, 1977, vol. 3,№ 5, c. 18-20.
106. Skulachev V.P. Ratio of oxidation and phosphorylation in the respiratory chain. - Moscow: USSR Academy of Sciences, 1962, - 156 p.
107. Skulachev V.P. - Accumulation of energy in the cell. - M.: Nauka, 1969, -440 c.
108. Skulachev V.P. - Energy transformation in biomembranes. - M.: Nauka, 1972, - 204 p.
109. Sologub G.R., Demidenko N.M., Izmailova G.D. Influence of pesticides on oxidative phosphorylation and activity of some enzymes of liver mitochondria. - In Collection: Scientific-research works of the Central Scientific Research Centre of Medical Universities of Uzbekistan. Samarkand, 1974, vol. 2, p. 109.
110. Staples R, Kellam R, Heisman J. Development of toxic effects in rats during pregnancy after feeding or gastric administration of the organophosphorus pesticides dipterex and imidan. - In the book: Mater. I final Soviet-American Symp. on the problem: "Environmental Hygiene", Riga, M.: Medicine, 1975, p. 163-172.
111. Toropova G.P., Egorov E.V. Changes in the content of nucleic acids in tissues and liver nuclei of white rats under chlorophos exposure. - Questions of Nutrition, 1967, te I, p. 16-20.
112. Trefilov V.N., Fayerman I.S. Labour conditions and state of health of workers in the production of dust, metaphos. - Hygiene and Sanitation, 1965, No. 2, p. 109-!!!-.
113. Khakimov 3.3., Najimutdinov K.N., Kamilov I.K. Effect of HCHCG, butifos, TMTD on the content of proteins, glycogen and total lipids in the liver. - Questions of Pharmacology and Pharmacy, 1973, p. 246-251.
114. Hakimov 3.3., Najimutdinov K.N., Kamilov I.K. Indicators of energy metabolism of the liver in acute intoxication with pesticides. - In Collected Works: Pharmacol. and Toxicol. Tashkent, 1973, p. 100-104.
115. Khakimov 3.3., Nadzhimutdinov K.N., Sologub G.R. Some of the

Biochemical parameters of energy metabolism of rat liver during long-term administration of butifos in low doses. - In Collected Works: Problems of Pharmacol. and Toxicol. Tashkent, 1975, p. 87-92.
116. Khalikov T.S., Agzamov X., Gulyamov T.D., Almatov K.T. Study of the effect of bazudin on carbohydrate-lipid metabolism in the liver of rats. - In book: Theses of reports of the U1 All-Union conf. "Problems of hygiene and toxicology". Kiev: Naukova Dumka, 1981, Part P, p. I40-141.
117. KhamidovD .Kh., KhakimovP .A., ShaikhovR. T.
Luminescence-chemical analysis of hepatocytes of developing embryos in ontogenesis. - Dokl. of the Academy of Sciences of the Uzbek SSR, 1174, No.6, p.54-56.
118. Khamidov D.H., Mirahmedov A.K., Sheraliev A.. Functional activity of liver mitochondria of embryos and maternal organism under the action of butifos. - In the collection: Mater. All-Union symposium "Stress, adaptation and functional disorders". Kishinev, Shtin-tsa, 1984, p.239.
119. Heisin E.M. Normal and pathological cytology of parenchyma. L.: Nauka, 1960, p.68-71.
120. Khuriev B.B., Gofmekler V.A., Danilov V.B. About some indicators of embryotropic action of methylmercaptophos in experiment. - In Collection: Mater, scientific-practical conf. of Resp. society of pathological anatomists of Uzbekistan. Tashkent: Medicine, 1969, p.51-53.
121. Tsapko V.G.Mate[л] ly on toxicogogy and hygienic normisation of chlorophos. - Avtoref.kand.kand.dis...biol. sciences, 1965, - 21 p.
122. Shabarchin E.I., Kruglyakova K.E., Handel L.Ya. On the possibility of using biological membranes as models for evaluation of biological activity of pesticides. - Dokl.AS USSR, 1977, vol. 234, №2, c.490-492.
123. Shabarchin E.I., Kruglyakova K.E., Handel L.Y., Kabanov V.V.
Study of the effect of metaphos on the structural and functional organisation of mitochondrial membranes. - Izv. of the USSR Academy of Sciences, ser.biol. 1979, No.6, p.937-942.
124. Sheraliev A., Almatov K.T., Mirahmedov A.K. Action of butifosan activity of polyenzyme systems of mitochondria membranes of liver mitochondria of foetus and pregnant rabbits.- Uzbek.biol.zhurnal, 1984, №2, p.42-44.
125. Sheraliev A. Study of tissue and subcellular distribution of konton (fluomethiuron) and butifos through the placenta at late gestation of rats. Scientific Bulletin of NamSU 2019,No. 10, pp. 123-128.
123 Sheraliev A., Otamirzaev Sh., Shukurjonov M. The effect of butifos on the number of phospholipid lysoforms of mitochondrial membranes of rabbit liver mitochondria in embryogenesis. "Actual problems of fundamental sciences of physiology and valeology ", Republican Scientific Online Conference Namangan, 2020, June, p. 78-80. 78-80.
124 Shvets V.I., Glebov R.N., Tolstikova G.V. Ability of lipids to reactivate ia,K-

ATPase of rat brain. - $d_{окл}$. dts USSR, 1974, vol.217, No.3, pp.733-735.
125 .Abo-Khatwa N., Hollingworth R.M. Pesticidal chemicals affecting some energy-linked functions of rat liver mitochondria in vitro. - Bull. Environ. Contam.& Toxicol. 1974, v. 12,No. 4, p. 446-454.
126 .Askermann H.Ubergang phosphororganischer Insectizide in den Embryo-Biidung der Po-Derivate und Auslosung toxisch- er Symptome.- Tag,, Acad. Landvir-tseh.-Wiss., GDR, Berlin, 1974, v. 126, p.23-29.
126 .Ackrell B.A.C.,Kearney E.B.,Merli A.,LudwigB.,Capaldi A. Interactions between succinate dehydrogenase and its membrane environment.- Mech. Oxid.Enzymes., Amsterdam e®a., 1978, p.143-154.
127 .Agranoff B.W.. Biochemicol mechanisms in the phosphofidyl- inositol effect. Neurosci. Lab., Vniv.of Michigan, 1103 East Huron Ann Arbor , M I 48109, US , Life Sci., 1983,v. 32,N18, p. 20472054.
128 . Anderson E.,Condon W.,Sharp D.. A study of oogenesis in
the rabbit Oryctolagus cuniculus with specific reference to the structural changes mitochondria.- J. Morphol.,1970, v.130, N1, p.67-91 o
129 . Aprille I.R.. Net uptake of adenine nucleotides by newborn rat liver mitochondria.- Arch. Biochem and biophys. 1981,N1, p.157-164.
130 . Augustin W.,Zborowski J.,Baranska J.,Wiswedel I., Wojte- zak L.- Synthesis of phospholipids in mitochondria and other membrane fractions of rabbit reticulocytes.- Bio- chim,biophys.acta., 1977, v#483, N2, p.298-306.
131 .Augustini Cx's.ns iF.Xi. Ac uxon of phospholipase A on mitochondrial cristal. Biochim, et biophys.acta.,1969, v.189, N3, p.457-461.
132 .Awasthi Y.C.,Chuang T.P.,Keenan T.W.,Crane PcL. Association of cardiolipin and cytochrome oxidase.- Biochem,Biophys. Res. Communs, 1970, ve39, N5, p.822-832.
133 .Awasthi Y.C.,Chuang T.F.,Keenan T.W.,Crane P.b.- Tightly- bound cardiolipin in cytochrome oxidase.- Biochim.biophys. acta. 1971, ve226, N1, p.42-53.
134 .Bababunmi EoAo,01orunsogo 0.0.,Bassir 0. The uncoupling effect of N-(phosphonomethyl) glycine on isolated rat liver mitochondria.- Biochem.pharmacol., 1979, v.28, N6, p.925- 927.
135 .Baginski E.S.,Poa P.P.,2ak B. Microdetermination of inorganic phosphate,phospholipids and total phosphate in biologic meters. Clin.chem.acta, 1967, v.13, N9, p.326-332.
136 Baranska W.,Dorywalski K.,Szymkowiak W.. Ultrastructural and sterological investigation of mitochondria in the pre- iplantation stage of mouse embryo development.- Ann.Med. SecoAcad.Sci., 1976, v.21, N2, p.13-14.
137 . Bereziat G. Renouvellement des asides gras des membranes cellalaires. Ann.nutr et alim, 1980, v.34, N2, p.241-254.
138 .Berezney R.,Awasthi Y.C,Crane PoL. The relation of phospholipid and membrane-bounol ATPase in mitochondrial electron transport particles. J.Bioenerget. 1970, v.1, N5,.p.457-465".

139. Bisson R;Montecucco C.,Gutweniger H.,Azzi A. Cytochrome~c~ oxidase subunits in contact with phospholipids "Hydrophobic photolabelling with azidophospholipids.- J.Biol.Chem. 1979, v.254, N20, p.9962-9965.
140.Bonini R.I.C.,Alonso T.S.,Bazan S.G. Phosphatidic acid, phosphatidylinositol,phosphatidylserine and cardiolipid in the course of early embryonic development.Patty acid composition and contre in whole toad embryos and mitochondrial fractions. Biochim.biophys.acta. 1981, v.664, N3, p. 561-571.
141. Bremer J., Greenberg D.M. Methyl transferring enzyme system of microsomes in the biosynthesis of lecithin (phos- phatidilcholine). - Biochim.Biophys. Acta, 1961, v. 46, No. 2, p. 205-216.
142. Brierley G©P., Merola A., Fleischer S. Studies of the electron transfer system. 49. Sites of phospholipid involvement in the electron-transfer chain. - Biochim. Biophys. Acta, 1962, v. 64, Noo 2, po 218-228.
143.Bruni A., Racker E.'Resolution and reconstitution of the mitochondrial electron transport system. - J. Biol. Chem., 1968, v. 243, no. 5, p. 962-971.
144.Bruni A., Toffano G. Lisophosphosphatidylserine a short-lived intermediate with plasma membrane regulatory properties© - Pharmacol. Res. Communs, 1982, v. 14, No. 6, p. 469-484.
145. Budreau C.H., Singh R.P. Teratogenecity and embryotoxicity of demefon and fenthion in CK-1 mouse embryos. - Toxicol. Appl. Pharmacol., 1973" v. 24, No. 2, p. 324-332.
146. Cabo-Soler J., Sechi A.M., Parenti-Castelli G., Lenaz G.. Inadequacy of myelin phospholipids for restoration of suc- cinooxidase activity in lipid-depleted mitochondria. - J. Bioenerget., 1971, v. 2, no© 2, p. 129-134.
147. Chan S.H., Higgins E. Uncoupling activity of endogenous free fatty acids in rat liver mitochondria. - Canad. J. Biochem., 1978_r $v.56_3$ Ho. 2S p. 111-116"
148.Chance B., V/illiams J.M. The respiratory chain and oxidative phosphorylation. - Advan. Enzymol., 1956, v. 17, no. 1, p. 65-135.
149.Chedid A., Nair V. Ontogenesis of cytoplasmic organelles in rat hepatocytes and the effect of prenatal phenobarbital on endoplasmic reticulum development# - Develop. Biol., 1974, v. 39, No. 1, p. 49-62.
150. Chuang ChoCh., Oliver J.T.. Role of adenosine cyclic monophosphate in the synthesis of tyrosine aminotransferase in neonatal rat liver.
Release of enzyme from membrane-borug polysomes in vitro. - Biochemistry, 1971, v. 10, No. 16, p. 2990-3001.
151.Chuang T.F., Awasti Y.C., Crane F.L.. The model mosaic cytochrome oxidase membrane. - In: Abstr. 54th Ann. Meeting in Atlantic Cityc Federat.Proc., 1970, v. 29, p 540.
152.Chuang T.F., Crane P.L.. Phospholipids in the cytochrome oxidase reaction. - J. Bioenerget, 1973 v. 4, No. 6, p. 563- 578.
153. Danseu G.P, Shapiro B.M The HADH dehydrogenase of the respiratory chain of Escherichia coli. II. Kinetics of the purified enzyme.- J. Biol. Chem., 1976, v. 251, No.

19, p. 5921-5928.
154.Di Francesco C., Brodbeck U.Interaction of human red cell membrane acetylcholinesterase with phospholipids. - Biochim. Biophys. Acta, 1981, v. 640, no. 1, p. 359-364.
155.Duck-Chong G.G., Poliak J.K.. - In: The Biochemistry of gene expression in urgher organism. - Austr. & New Zeeland Book Publishing Co., Sydney, 1973,p. 305.
156.Erecinska M., Wilson D. F., Miyata Y. Mitochondrial cytochrome b~c-- complex: its oxidation-reduction components and their stoichiometry. - Arch. Biochem.Biophys., 1976, v.177,No. 1, p. 133-143.
157. Ernster L., Dalner G., Azzone G.P. Differential effects of rotenone and amital on mitochondrial electron and energy
Transfer. - J. Biol. Chem., 1963, v0 238, No. 2, p. 1124- 1131.
158. Ernster b., Kuylenstiema B. Outer membrane of mitochondria. - In: Membranes of mitochondria and chloroplasts. (Van Nostrand & Reinhold - Eds.). N.Y., 1970, p. 172-212o
159. Fain J.N.,Liu Suc-Hwa,Litosch I.,Wallace M. Hormanal regulation of phosphatidylinositol brean down.- Life Sci , 1983, v. 32, N8, p. 2055-2067.
160. Pelter S.A.,Stahi A. Properties of a hydrophobic protein from yeast mitochondria inner memdrane.- Biochimie, 1978, v. 60, N10, p. 1175-1199. 1175-1179.
161. Peo P.,Canuto R.A.,Garcea R.,Brossa 0. The role of lipid- protein interactions in NAD.H-cytochrome-c-reductase (ro- tenone-insensitive) of rat liver mitochoodria.- Biochem.biophys.actao 1978, v. 504, N1, p. 1-14.
162. Fish S.A. Organophosphorus cholinesterase inhibitors and fetal development.- Amer. J.obstet. Gynecol. 1966, v. 96, N8, p. 1148-1154.
163. Fleischer S.,Klouwen H. The role of soluble lipid in mitochondrial enzyme sustem.- Biochem.and Biophys. Res Communs, 1961, v. 5, N5, p. 378-383.
164. Fleischer S.,Casu A.,Pleischer B.. A phospholipid reguire- ment for NADH oxidation in mitochondria.- Ital.J.Biochem,
1977, v. 26, N4, p. 277-296.
165. Folch Pi.J.,Lees M.,Sloane-Stanley G.H.. Asimple method
for the isolation and purification of total lipids of animal tissues.- J.Biol.Chem. 1957, v. 226, N1, p. 497-509.
166. Fry M.,Green D.E.. Cardiolipid reguirement by cytochrome
oxidase and the catalytic role of phospholipid.- Biochem.
and Biophys. Res. Commun. 1980, v.93, N4, p.1238-1246.
167. Fry M., Green D. Cardiolipin reguirement for elektron fras- fer in complex I and III of the mitochondrial respiratory chain.- J.Biol.Chem. 1981, v.256, N4,p.1874-1880.
172. Fry M., Green D.E.. Studies on the resolution of cytochrome oxidase.- J.Bioenerg.and Biomembr. 1981, v.13, N1-2, p. 61- 87.
173. Gan-Elepano M., Mead J.F.. The function of phospholipase Ag in them

metabolism of membrane lipids.- Biochem. Biophys.Res. Communs., 1978, v.89, N1, p.247-251.
174. Gazzotti P. Mitochondria: a general survey..- Top. Bioelec- trochem and Bioenergeties.- 1980, v.3, P" 149-190.
175. Gericke C., Hettwer H., Staib W. Changes in fatty acid pattern of plasma membranes and of mitochondria in rat liver after poisoning with organophosphates.- Biochem. Exp. Biol., 1976, v.12, N3, p. 293-305.
176. Gibson K.D., Wilson J.D., Udenfriend S. The Enzymatic Conversion of Phospholipid Ethanolamine to Phospholipid Choline in Rat liver.- J.Biol.Chem, 1961, v.236,N3,p.673-679.
177. Godinot C. Nature and Possible Function of Associtiion bat- ween Glutamate Dehydrogenase and Cardiolipin.- Biochemistry, 1973, v.12, N21, p.4029-4034.
178. Greenfield P.C., Boell E.J.. Succinic dehydrogenase and cytochrome oxidase of mitochondria of chick liver and skeletal muscle during embryonic development. - J.Exper.Zool., 1968, v. 168, p.491-500.
179. Hallman M. Changes in mitochondrial respiratory chain proteins during prenatal development of enviromental oxygentension.- Biochim,biophys. acta.1971,v.253,N2, p.360-372.
180. Hallman M., Kanlare P. Cardiolipin and cytochrome AA3 in inta et liver mitochondria of rats. Evidence of successive formation of inner membrane components.- Biochem.Biophys. Res. Communs. 1971,v.45, N4, p.1004-1110.
181. Hatefi Y., Haavik A.G., Grffiths D.E.. Studies on the electron transport system.- J.Biol.Chem. 1962, v.237, N5,p.1681-1685.
182. Hathwoy D.E., Amoroso E.C. The effects of pesticides on mam- mali an reproduction.- Toxicol.Biodegradet. and Effic. Livestock Pesticides, Amsterdam,1972, p.213-251.
183. Hettwer H., Gericke Ch. Lipide der Plasma membrane und der Mitochondrien ans Rattenlever nach Paraoxon-IntexsKation.- Arch.Toxicol.,1977,v.38, N4, p.251-260.
184. Hundt E., Kadenbach B. On the molecular weight of mitochon- drially aynthesised subunits of rat liver cytochrome oxidase. J.Physiol.Chem, 1977,v.358, N10, p.1309-1314.
185. Hunter D.R., Komai N., Haworth R.A. Oxidative phospholytion and respiratory control in lysolecithin treated electron transport particles. - Biochem.Biophys. Res.Communs, 1974, v,56, N3, p.647-653.
186. . Ivanetich K.M.,Henderson J. J.,Kaminsky L.S.-Some properties of a cytochrome-c-mixed mitochondrial phospholipid Complex.- Biochemistry, 1974,v.13,N6,p.1469-1476.
187. Kadenbach B. Synthesis of mitochondrial proteins: Demonstrations of a transfer of proteins from microsomes into mitochondria. -Biochem. biophys.acta.1967,v.134,N2,p.430-442.
188. Kandas Wami C.,D'Lorio A. On rat liver mitochondrial mono

amine oxidase activity and lipids.-Arch.Biochem.biophys, 1978,v.190, N2, p.847-849.
189. Keranen A.,Kankare P.,Hallman M. Changes of fatty acid composition of phospholipids in liver mitochondria and microso- mea of the during grouth.-Lipids, 1982,v.17,N3,p.155-159^
190. Kimbrough R.,Gaines T. Effect of organic phosphorus compounds adn alkylating agents on the fetus.-Arch.Environ. Health, 1968,v.16, p.805808.
191. 'Kleinrok Z., Jagiello-V/ogtowicz E.,Sieklucka~Dziuba M. - Effects of fluorostignine,toxogonin and atropine on monoamine oxidase activity and the level of biogenie amines in mouse brain.- Acta physiol.pol.,1979,v.30.N4.P.437-444.
192. Kolorav J.,Wielburski A.,I.B.Mendel-Hartvig, B.D.Nelson. Synthesis of cytochrome oxidase in isolated rat hepatocytes.- Biochem.biophys.acta,1981,v.652,N2, p.334-346.
193. Laley B.O.,Gibson M.A. Association of hipogbycemia and pancreatic leiet tissul with micromelia and malformation treated chick embryos. - Can.J.Zool.,1977,v.55,N2,p.261-264.
194. Lamboni L.Mastrojanni L.Electron microscopic studies on rabbit ova.- J.Ultrast.Res.1966,v.14,N1,p.95-117.
195. Lardy H.A.,Welman H.Oxidative phosphorylation: Role of inorganic phosphate and acceptor system in control of metabolic
J.J.Biol.chem., 1952,v. 185, p.215.
196. Lee C.P. A fluorescent probe of the hydrogen ion concentration in ethylendinetetzacetic acid particles of beef mitochondria. -Biochemistry, 1971,v.10,N10, p.4375-4381.
197. Lenas G.,Ca3telli A.,Littarru G.P.,Bertoli E.,Folkers K.Spec- ificity of lipids and coenzyme Q in mitochondrial NADH and suce
cin-oxidase of Beet Heart and S.cerevisiae. 1971, v.142,N2,p.407-416.
198. Levy M.,Toury R.,Sauner M.T.,Andre J. Recent findings of the biochemical and enzymatic composition of the tab isolated mitochondrial membranes in relation to their structure.- PEBS Sympos, 1960, v.17, pc 33-42.
199. Linda Yu.,Chang-An Vy King T.E.. Subunit structure of the re- constitutively active cytochrome b-c, compleXoDetermination of amine acids and molar distribution of subunit fraction from gel electrophoresis.- Biochim.Biophys.Acta. 1977. v. 495,N2, p. 232-247.
200. Lowry O.H.,Rosebrough W.I.,Farr A.L.,Randell R.I. Protein measurement with the folin phenol resgent.-Jo biol.chem., 19510 vc139f N1, p.265-275.
201. Lutz-Oslertog Y.,Heiniel R.,Sutz H. Effect du paration sur le developmenthment de l.embryon de caille et de certains de ses organes in "vivo" et in "vitro".- Bull.biol.Prance et Belgiguf, 1969, v.103, N3, P. 468-470.
202. Machinist J.M.,Singer T.P.,Reaction of coenzyme Q in the DPNH dehudrogenase segment of the respiratory chain.-Proc.Nat. Acad. Sci. USA., 1965, v.53. N2, p, 467-474.
203. Mackler B.,Grace R.,Duncan H.M. Studies of mitochondrial development

during embryogenesis in the rat.- ArcheBiochem. Biophys. 1971.v.144, N23. p. 603-610.

204. Maisterrena B.,Comte J.,Gantheron D.C. Purification of pig heart mitochondrial membranes. Enzymatic and morphological characteisation as cmpared to microsomes.- Biochem. Biophys. Acta, 1974, v. 367, N2, p. 115128.

205. Marfson L.V.,Voronina V.M. Experimental sfudy of the effect of a series of phosphororganic pesticides (dipterex and imi- dan) on embryogenesis.- Environ.HealthePerspect, 1976, v.13, p. 121-125.

206. Masliuska D.,Zalewska Z. Effect of dichlophos administred to the pregeny. Polia histochem. cytochem. 1978, v. 16,N4, p. 334-341.

207. McMurray M.C., Magee W.L.. Phospholipid metabolism. - Ann.
Revo Biochem., 1972, v. 41, p. 129-160.

208. Nakazawa T., Asami E., Suzuki H., Yukawa 0o Appearence of energy coservation system in rat liver mitichondria during development. The role of adenine nucleotide translocation.
68. J. Biochem. 1973. v. 73. No. 2, p. 397-406.

209. Neville D.M., Clossmanh H. Plasma membrane protein subunit composition. A comparative study by discontinuous electrophoresis in sodium dodecyl sulfate. - J. Biol. Chem., 1971, v. 246, no. 20, p. 6335-6338.

210. Nishibayashi Y.H.,Cunningham C.C., Racker E. Resolution and reconstitution of mitochondrial electron transport system. III. Order of reconstitution and requirement for a new factor for respiration. - J. BIOL. Chem., 1972, v. 247, No. 3, p. 698-704.

211. O'Brien P., Matlid A., Organisation of the citric acid cycle enzymes in the mitochondrial matrix. - (9th Int. Cong. Biochem., Stokholm, 1973). Abstr. Book, Stokholm, 1973.P. 378.

212. OLORUNSOGO O., Bababunmi E. A., Bassir O. The inhibitory effeet
of N-(phosphomonomethyl)-glicine in vivo on energy-dependent phosphate-induced swelling of isolated rat liver mitochondria. - Toxicol. Lett., 1979, v. 4, p. 303-306.

213. Parce J.W., Cunningham C.C., Waite M. Mitochondrial phospho-.
Lipase A2 activity and mitochondrial aging. - Biochemistry,
1978, v. 17, no. 9, p. 1634-1639.

214. Parenti-Castelli G., Sechi A.M., Landi L., Cabrim L., Nascarello S., Lenaz G.. Lipid-protein interaction in mitichond- ria. VII. A comparison of the effect of lipid removal and lipid perturbation on the kinetic properties of mitochondrial ATPase. - Biochim. Biophys.Acta, 1979, v. 547, N1, p. 161169.

215. Parsons S.P., Simsons M.Y.. Biosynthesis of DNA by isolated mitochondria. Incorporation of thymidine triphosphate - 2- C^{14} . - Science, 1967, v. 155, N 3758, p. 91-93.

216. Pitotti A., Dabbeni-Sola P., Bruni A. Phospholipid-depen- dent assembly of mitochondrial ATPase complex. - Biochim. Biophys. Acta, 1980, v. 600,n1, p. 78-80.

217. Poliak J.Ko, Woog Mo Changes in proportions of two mitochondrial

populations during the development of embryonic chick liver. - Biochem. J., 1971, v. 123, N. 3, P.347-353.
218. Poliak J.K.. The maturation of the inner membrane of foetal rat liver mitochondria. An example of a positive-feedback mechanism. - Biovhem. J., 1975, ve 150o N. 3, P. 477-488.
219. Poliak J.K., Sutton R. The transport and accumulation of adenine nucleotides during mitochondrial biogenesis. - Biochem. J., 1980, v. 192, N. 1, p. 75-83.
220. Poyton R.O., Schaftz G. Cytochrome-c-oxidase from bakers
yeast. III. Physical characterisation of isolated subunits and chemical evidence for two different classes of polypep- tides$_0$ - J. Biol. Chem., 1975, v. 250, N. 2, p. 752-76l.
221. Proctor N.H., Casida E. Organophosphorous and methyl carbomate insecticide teratogenesis: diminished NAD in chicken embryos. - Science, 1975, v. 190, N 4214, p. 580-582.
222. Racker E - Mechanisms in bioenergetics.- N.Y.-London,
Acad. Press, 1975, - 259 p.
223. Raw L., Makler H.R.. Studies of electron transport enzymes.,J. Biol. Biol. Chem., 1959, v. 234, N 7, p. 1867-1873.
224. Rosas S.B., Carmen S.M., Ghittoni V©E. Effect of pesticides on the fatty acids and phospholipid composition of Es~ chericia coli. - Appl. & Environ. Microbiol., 1980, v. 40,N 2, Po 231-234.
225. Rydstrom J., Kanner N., Racker E. - Biochem.Bipphys. Res. Communs, 1975. v. 67, p. 831-839.
226. Schatz G., Mason T.L.The biogenesis of mitochondrial proteins. - Ann. Rev. Biochem., 1974, v. 43, N 1, p. 51~87.
227. Schnaitman C.A., Greenwald I.M. Enzymatic properties of the inner and outer membranes of rat liver mitochondria. - J. Cell. Biol., 1968, v. 38, p. 158-175.
228. Schnaitman C.A., Greenwald I.M. Further studies on the localisation of enzymes in mitochondria. - J. Cell. Biol., 1968, v. 35, p. 254-260.
229. Schneider W.C., Hogeboom GoH.Intracellular distribution of enzymes. V. Further studies on the distribution of cytochrome c in rat liver gomogenates. - J. Biol. Chem., 1950, v.p. 123-131.
230. Scholte H. R. The separation and enzymatic characterisation of inner and outer membranes of rat heart mitochondria. - Biochim. Biophys. Acta, 1973, v. 330, N 3, p. 283-293.
231. Sebald W., Machleidt W. Otto J. Products of mitochondrial protein synthesis of Neurospora crassa.Determination of equimolar amounts of three products in cytochrome oxidase on the basis of amino acid analysis. - Eur. J. Biochem., 1973, v. 38, N 1, p. 311-324.
232. Seits H.J., Muller M.J., Krone W, Tarnowski W. Coordinate control of intermediary metabilism in rat liver by the insulin/glucagon ratio during stakvation and after glucoserefeeding. - Arch. Biochem. Biophys, 1977, v. 183, N2, p. 647-663.
233. Shud A.L., Shrago E., Bittar N., Folts J.D., Koke JoR.Acyl-CoA inhibition of

adenine nucleotide translocation in ischemic myocardium. - Amer. J. Physiol., 1975, v. 228, J 3, p. 689-692.
234. Sitkewicz D., Zalewska Z. Effect of organophosphate insecticides on some oxidoreductase in rat brain mitochondria. - Neuropathol.Pol., 1975, v. 13, N 3-3, p. 4-63-469.
235. Sitkewicz D., Konecka A.M., Chojnocka-Baldys K. Czhych naoktywnose oskydazycytochromowej i dehydrogenazy bursztynia- nowej mozgy szczura i kury. - Rocz.Panet.Zakl.nig., 1976,3, P. 277-286.
236. Sirkewcz D., Skonieczna M., Ortowska E., Bicz W.The effect of organophosphorous insecticides on the oxidative processes in rat brain mitochondria.Comparative studies of chlorfen- vinphos and its chemical analodse - Weuropathol.polo, 1978, v. 16., N 4, p. 487-495.
237. Sjostrand P.S. The structure of mitochondrial membranes: a new concept. - J. Ultrastruc. Res., 1978, v. 64, N 3, P. 217-245.
238. Skonieczna M., Weirciak M., Scislowska I., Biez W. Influence of chlorfenvinphos and ipophos on oxidoreduction processes in rat brain mitichondria during development. - Neuro- patol. pol., 1981, v. 19, N 2, p. 197-208.
239. Smoly J.M., Kuylenstierna B., Ernster Lo Topological and functional organisation of the mitochondria. - Proc. Natl. Acad. Sci. USA, 1970, v. 66, N 1, p. 125-131.
240. Spetale M.R., Moricoli LoS., Rodriguez G.E.. The effect oforganophosphorous compounds on respiration by rat liver mitochondria. - Farmacol. Ed. Sci., 1977, v. 32, N 2, p. 166-172.
241. Staples R.S., Kellam R.G., Haseman J.K.. Developmental toxicity in the rat after injection or gavage of organophosphorous pesticides (dipterex, imidan) during pregnancy. - Environ. Health.Respect., 1976, v. 13, p. 133141.
242. Staszyc J. Kifer Eo,Badania nad vpliwen preparatu foafor- organicznego na organizm ciczanyck szczucow i plodov oraz na Komorki w Holowki tranlowej. - Ann UMCS, 1974, D 29, p. 249-254.
243. Stephans R.J., Bils R.P. Ultrastructural changes in developing chick liver. I. General cutology. - J. Ultrastruct.
Rs., 1967, v. 38., N 3, p. 456-474.
244. Stoffel W., Schniefer H.G.. *3C-nuclear magnetic resonance studies of lipid interactions in single and multicomponent lipid vesicles. - J. Phys. Chem., 1968, v. 349, N 23, p. 1097.
245. Swirczynski J., Scislowski P., Aleksandrowicz Z. High activity of - glycerophosphate oxidation by human placental mitochondria. - Biochim. Biphys. Acta, 1976, v. 429, I 1, p. 46-54.
246. Szarkowska L. The restoration of DPKH oxidase activity by coenzyme Q (ubiquinone). - Afch. Biochem. &Biophys., 1966, v. 113, N 3, p. 519-525.
247. Thompson E.D., Parks L.W.. Lipid associated with cytochrome
Oxidase derived from yeast mitochondria. - Biochim. Biophyso Acta, 1972, v. 260, N

2, p. 601-607.
248. Tos-Luty S., Puchla W., Latuszynska J. Badaia toksysznos- cichlorfenvinfosu dla zaradkow kurrych. -Bromatol. i chem. toksycol.,1972, v.5, *J,* P.339-343.
249. Vignais P.V. Molecular and physiological aspects of adenine nucleotide transport in mitochondria. Biochim.Biophys.Acta, 1976, v.456, N1,p.1-38.
250. Virji M., Knowles P. Protein-lipid interactions in cytochrome oxidase firrom S. serevisiae. Effects of detergents and reconstitution of enzyme activity by phospholipids by using cholate mediated exchange.- Biochem. J.,1978, v.169, N2, p.343-350.
251. Yeung D., Oliver J.T.. Factors affecting the premature induction of phosphopiruvate carboxylase in neonatal rat liver. Biochem. J.,1968, v.108, N2, p.325-331.
252. Wharton D.C.,GriffethsD.E.. Assay of cytochrome oxidase effect of phospholipids and other factors.- Arch. Biochem. Biophys., 1961, v.96, N1,p.103-114.
253. Weiss H., Juchs B. Isolation of a multiprotein complex con- ' taining cytochrome b and c from Neurospora crassa mitochondria by affinity chromatography on immobilised cytochrome e and ferrocytochrome c to the multiprotein complex. - Eur. J.Biochem.,1978, v.88,$T 1, p.17-28.
254. Wilson J.C. Amer.j.Anatom., 1973, v.136, N6.
255. Zanler W., Fleischer S.J.. Kinetic studies of the lipid requirement of mitochondrial cytochrome c oxidase. - J.Bio- energet., 1971, v.2, N 3-4, p.209215.

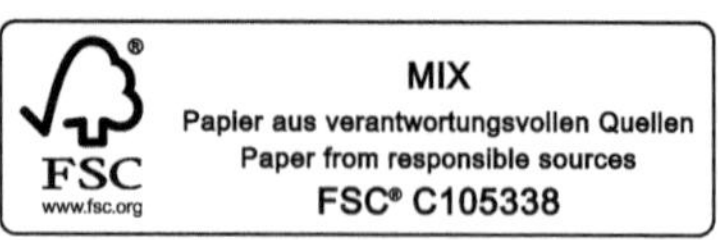

Printed by Books on Demand GmbH, Norderstedt / Germany